THE HALF A MILLION POUND GIRL

THE HALF A MILLION POUND GIRL

SARAH BURGE

WITH DEREK CLEMENTS

FOREWORD BY ALLEY EINSTEIN

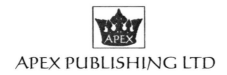

APEX PUBLISHING LTD

First published in 2011 by
Apex Publishing Ltd
PO Box 7086, Clacton on Sea, Essex, CO15 5WN

www.apexpublishing.co.uk

British Library Cataloguing-in-Publication Data
A catalogue record for this book
is available from the British Library

ISBN 1-906358-88-5
978-1-906358-88-4

Typeset in 10pt Baskerville Win95BT

Production Manager: Chris Cowlin

Photos: Supplied by the author

Printed and bound by
MPG Books Group in the UK

Publishers Note:
The views and opinions expressed in this publication are those of the author and are not necessarily those of Apex Publishing Ltd

Copyright:
Every attempt has been made to contact the relevant copyright holders,
Apex Publishing Ltd would be grateful if the appropriate people contact us on:
01255 428500 or mail@apexpublishing.co.uk

Sarah Burge's website: **www.thesarahburge.com**

To my husband Tony, where life began and where it will end.
Without you there would be no story.

To Charlotte, Hannah and Poppy, my wonderful daughters. Life is one big adventure and I'm so glad to be sharing it with you. For all the loves I have had in my life, nothing comes close or compares to the love I have for you.

CONTENTS

ACKNOWLEDGEMENTS

Mum and Dad, Clara and Eric, for putting up with me all these years;

Tony's mother Pat, and his late father Edward, for always believing, that we were meant to be together;

My late brother Trevor, whom we still miss terribly – a constant source of inspiration who mostly played the bad guy in films but to me will always be the good guy;

Jasmine Burge, you will always be like a daughter to me;

Ruthann and the boys, Travis and Daniel, who would make their Dad truly proud;

Ann Goody, Margaret, Ian and Eric, for the fun we have shared;

Richard Glynn, the first media mogul to help me launch my career, www.thebuzzfactory.co.uk;

Martin Marshall, my most trusted friend, colleague, brilliant photographer and film-maker. We have laughed until we dropped. His pictures appear on the cover and inside this book, www.wix.com/morosart/moro;

Paul Webb, friend and photographer whose pictures appear in this book, www.pwebb.co.uk;

Neil Kingston, presenter/creative director who gave his time and talent to help me, www.neilrobertkingston.co.uk;

The late Andrew Savage, a make-up artist whose talents were beyond his years;

Amanda Linke, my fabulous make-up artist extraordinaire, amandalinke@biscituk.com;

Grant Hayes, for all your love and wit.

Karen, Carmel, Kim, my three most trusted long-term friends, seeing me through the good, the bad and the most ugly of times;

Claire Jennings, my dearest friend and confidante. We are but the same!

Lesley, Beth, Bonnie, Laura, Justine, Vicky, Melissa, Sophie, Kim, to name but a few of the fabulous mums of the children at Godmanchester Primary School, who stood by me and chose not to listen;

Amiee and Dan, whom I trusted with my most treasured little person;

Lee and Ryan Essex, by far my favourite paparazzi guys, www.isoimagesuk.com;

Mark Moody of OK! magazine for all the amazing parties we created;

Alley Einstein, for writing my foreword. A trusted friend and journalist who helped bring about the Sarah Burge Brand, www.alleyeinstein.co.uk;

Derek Clements, no words can express my thanks for all the hard work you put into helping me with this book;

Chris Cowlin, for giving me the opportunity to really tell it how it was and is;

And to everybody who has played a part in my life and helped to make me the person I am today.

My life is one big adventure and I live it to the full. I teach my children that life is a big adventure, too, and that they need to live, love and cherish every moment because before long you will blink and it will be gone.

Love, Sarah – a never-ending story.

FOREWORD

When I first met Sarah Burge or as many of you know her the Human Barbie I assumed she'd be a vacant air head obsessed with beauty with nothing between her ears. I expected when I asked how was she, to hear nothing but vacuous chatter about her various surgeries and lots of blonde hair flicking.

Instead for once I was proven wrong. As a journalist I've interviewed world leaders, celebrities, royalty and normal folk. Everyone has a story to tell. I know now that' Sarah's story is more fascinating than most celebs and even a few world leaders.

Behind the veneer of plastic surgery, makeup and hair extension lies a woman who until know has been too frightened to reveal the real Sarah. The publicity she received as THE HUMAN BARBIE made the world think that's all she was. However scratching beneath the surface and after hundreds of emails and phone calls and meetings I discovered much more.

Sarah is a lioness of a mother. She adores her three children and yes controversially has made headlines in stories with them. However in her view like her the kids have to face the cameras and by opening up her home and telling the world what they get up to helps them cope better with celebrity and prepares them for business. Some say why? Others say Why Not.

I cried buckets the day I read Sarah's account of being a domestic abuse victim. This wasn't some made up tale but a real life experience she suffered at the hands of a former partner. Not many people know this about her. She hides it well. The beatings and rapes she endured were awful – no one deserves that. She was beaten to a pulp and it's why she started on the road to plastic surgery. Yes she admits she's a cosmetic surgery addict but along the way has help 1000's of other women make the correct plastic surgery choices.

She's a campaigner against domestic violence and freely gives her time to charity work to help sufferers. How many of us can say that. Yes she has also created the MADAME PINK persona and as you will read enjoys what some may say is a colourful sex life. Again I ask why? And she says Why not?

People like to put Sarah into the mad crazy bad mummy box. She is anything but that. She has seen it all, done it all and now has had the guts to put it down on paper. This book is a fantastic read and its revelations will stun some and shock others. I do hope if changes your mind about her but if it doesn't ask yourself "Why not". Ultimately this is a book about bravery, strength, betrayel, hope and the ability to find ones self in a world that is sometimes cruel and one sided.

If your a mum, a victim of domestic violence, have been bullied, castigated, or your interest in what lies behind the hype then this book is the book for you.

Sarah could have remained silent forever, but her desire is to help other women and men.

Sit down and re-live her life experiences at times tragic, horrific, joyous, and at times making her feel she was worthless.

Sarah is somebody we should draw inspiration from, and a battle to be heard, if she helps just one person Sarah has done her job.

Alley Einstein

Television and Radio Presenter and Journalist

www.apexpublishing.co.uk

CHAPTER ONE
Mirror, Mirror On The Wall ...

❝ Go on Sarah, take a look, I am certain you will be delighted with what we've done..." The bandages had been removed from my face and the nurse thrust a mirror into my hand, urging me to look at the surgeon's handiwork.

The problem was that I didn't want to look. All that I had ever had were my looks. But now they had been taken away from me. The man I had loved, the man I had loved and had wanted to spend the rest of my life with, had beaten the living daylights out of me. He had left my face in ruins, my confidence in tatters.

Before, I had revelled in the way I looked. I had used my appearance to get me through my life, but now I couldn't bear to see my reflection in a mirror. So I always turned my head the other way whenever I saw a mirror.

Somehow, I had allowed myself to be persuaded that the NHS could fix my nose. Deep down, I knew that the finished job wouldn't be what I wanted. And yet I had no choice. He had broken my nose so badly that it no longer looked like it belonged on my face. I didn't want it on my face.

Oh my God! How could I have been so stupid? How could I have put myself in a position where a man that I thought I loved, and who claimed to love me, could decide that no man would ever want to look at me again? How could any human being treat another as he did me?

Most of you will have been punched or kicked at some stage in your lives. One or two of you may even have been pushed down a flight of stairs. And I suppose it is inevitable that there are women out there who have suffered as I did on that fateful night.

Did you burn the dinner? Maybe it was too hot – or too cold. Or perhaps you looked at him the wrong way? Was it something that one of the children said? Or maybe it was your fault that the boss gave him a hard time at work? Or you didn't iron his shirt properly?

With me it was the dress. It was too short. I look back on it now and it still makes no sense to me whatsoever. He used to love it when I showed off my legs and my cleavage – and I used to love showing them off for him. For him. To him. Not to or for anybody else. But suddenly on that night I was a slag, a tart. And that was when the fists began to hit me, when the foot sank into my body...

And now here I was, recovering from an operation that I knew was going to be a disaster from the second that I agreed to have it. It was going to take more than an NHS nose job to put me back together again.

I had been beautiful before, until this animal got his hands on me. I could be beautiful once more, but not at the hands of a National Health Service surgeon. They saved lives, but they didn't save looks. They didn't do boob jobs or tummy tucks. They didn't do facelifts or silicone implants. And they definitely didn't do buttock implants.

Somewhere in the back of my mind an idea was beginning to stir. Plastic surgery, performed by the best that Harley Street has to offer – now that might just work. Paying for it might prove to be an obstacle, but I had overcome bigger ones in my life. Yes, that was the answer. I was sure that it was. Real-life Barbie, here I come.

"Go on Sarah, take a look, I am certain you will be delighted with what we've done..."

CHAPTER TWO
Evil Women

I was born in Croydon in 1960, and my brother Trevor came along two years later. My father is Eric Goddard and his wife is Claire.

My earliest memories are of Sidcup and Bromley. I still shudder at the thought of it, but I went to a convent school, where I was taught by nuns. To this day, I am not quite sure how I ended up going there because we were not Roman Catholics.

For a five-year-old girl, it was a pretty frightening experience. They say that your schooldays are meant to be the happiest of your life. Try telling that to the sisters. Almost without exception, they were cold-hearted, unfeeling women who seemed to enjoy inflicting pain and punishment upon innocent young children. They were evil sadists.

Not that I was especially innocent, even in those days. I always wanted to see how far I could push things. I was pretty good at school though, especially when it came to English. And whenever there was any chance of winning a prize, you would find me doing whatever I had to do to win. Even at that stage in my life, I was very competitive. I guess it is something that you are born with because it certainly wasn't something that either of my parents instilled in me. If I did something, I always wanted to do it properly.

I was precocious. If something had to be said, I was usually the one who had to say it, and not always at the right time. Rather than telling me, or my classmates, to be quiet, the nuns had their own way of keeping us in order – they would hit us over the knuckles with a ruler, or they would lock us in a cupboard. Nowadays they would be prosecuted for treating children in such a manner. They call it child cruelty, but back then it was called discipline.

You will not be surprised to learn that I ended up hating the nuns and everything that they stood for. Remember that these were women who had decided to pledge their lives to God. In truth, they were a bunch of frustrated old hags who shouldn't have been allowed with a million miles of a classroom full of children. They were wicked.

I remember being told that I asked too many questions. I am sorry? Isn't that precisely how children learn things?

"You are such an inquisitive girl Sarah. You ask far too many questions. We can't answer them."

"What do you mean, you can't answer them? Isn't that your job?"

A hand delivered across the back of my head would inform me that no, it wasn't their job.

The most obvious consequence of the way they treated me was that I hated religion from a very early age. I knew that these women were supposedly devoted to God, and I was certain that I didn't want anything to do with a religion that seemed to say it was okay to batter children with impunity.

It didn't take long before I found myself sitting and staring out of the classroom window, wishing that I was anywhere but there. If they couldn't, or wouldn't, answer me, what was the point of being there?

Funnily enough, the subject that they seemed most reluctant to discuss with us was religion. I was a little girl and I had heard all about God, but I wanted to know more – where was He? Who was He? The more I asked, the more annoyed they seemed to get. If they couldn't even talk to us about God, what hope did we have of ever learning anything from them? I made up my mind that he didn't exist. It was an awful time in my life.

The most bizarre thing of all was the Sunday service when we would all be forced to go to confession and own up to our sins. I just used to piss about. At that age I didn't know what sins were (I have more than made up for that since, as you will discover), so I just used to sit there and make things up. Sometimes the priest believed me, but more often than not he would see right through me and I would be in hot water again. I felt like Walter Mitty.

Remember that I wasn't even a Catholic, so I really didn't have the first idea of the significance of this process. Needless to say, my messing about used to lead to further punishment from the old hags.

You may wonder why I didn't go home and tell my parents about the way the nuns were treating us, but I suppose I was scared that my Dad might punish me as well if he thought I had been misbehaving in school.

My father was a Metropolitan Police detective and he had a great many contacts, one of whom had told him that St Mary's was a great school. I have various childhood memories of my father but the chief one was that he always seemed to be drunk. If you ever watched the series *Ashes To Ashes*, you will have an idea of what life with my father was like. My Dad was Gene Hunt. He was rude, he swore a lot, and he was always right. He was a big noise in the force, going on to became a chief inspector, and he was not a man to be messed with.

He worked with the drug squad and the fraud squad, and he used to go out drinking and come staggering back home at 3am. He used to come home and tell us some horrific stories. One that sticks in my mind relates to a woman who had been subjected to an especially vicious rape during which the man had got hold of an iron rod, stuck it inside her and caused her dreadful internal injuries. This was a story he related over the dinner table.

In saying that, he was generally good fun and he was a loving father who always had time for Trevor and I. He used to take us swimming and all the usual sort of stuff, but we had to accept that sometimes he had to work odd hours, so he wasn't always around.

And then there was the day he led a drugs bust on a house where John Lennon was living. He'd had a tip-off that there were drugs in the house and when they went in, Lennon and Yoko Ono were in bed making love. When Lennon realised what was going on, he offered Dad some money to make it go away but Dad refused.

The bust happened on 18 October, 1968. Dad led a team into Lennon's apartment in Montague Square in Marylebone. Two sniffer dogs were used and eventually a quantity of what turned out to be cannabis was found in a binocular case. Lennon and Ono were both arrested and taken to Paddington Green Police station and charged with possession of a banned substance and obstructing police. The charge of obstruction was later dropped, as was the possession of drugs against Ono, when John Lennon pleaded guilty to the charge.

Having been convicted of possessing drugs, Lennon was refused entry into the USA for some time – the irony, of course, is that had they extended the ban, Lennon would still be alive today. One of the officers who took part in the raid was Detective Sergeant Norman Pilcher, and Lennon later wrote a song after him called *The Pilcherman*.

It was a huge news story and the day after the arrest there was a picture on the front pages of the newspapers of my father leading one of the most famous men in the world towards a police car. My Dad. I couldn't believe it, and I was incredibly proud of him. He would eventually take early retirement from the police and set himself up as a car dealer in Lewisham.

Anyway, this man was hardly going to believe me if I told him the school he was sending me to was full of evil old crones, was he?

My brother ended up going there too. At one stage I decided to liberate Trevor from school. We didn't get very far – Sidcup High Street, I think.

I was a dreamer, and I used to spend time wandering around the local shops trying out make-up. I had seen my Mum putting on lipstick and I had seen all the glamorous women on television and in the movies, and I knew that I wanted to look like them. I don't know how, but even at that age I realised it was important to be able get boys interested in me.

After several years attending St Mary's we moved, and suddenly my life changed for ever. My new school, Pickhurst Junior, was a cesspit – there is no other word for it. I had been taught to speak properly, even having elocution lessons, and I suppose that I stuck out like a sore thumb when we moved because I thought the girls were all as rough as guts. They were dreadful, and I don't know why because the school was in a good area. Maybe they just felt that was the way they were supposed to act.

I didn't fit in at Pickhurst, and I was picked on. But I never let it get me down. I was determined that nobody was going to bully me, so I used to laugh at them and, by and large, it had the desired effect and they eventually left me to my own devices.

I got plenty of verbal abuse, but it was almost always because of the way I spoke. I gave as good as I got and in any event I wasn't too bothered about what the girls had to say because I found the boys far more interesting, and they didn't seem to be at all concerned about the way I spoke. Funny that, isn't it?

Needless to say, the girls didn't like me spending all my time with the boys either. I guess they felt threatened, which was utterly ridiculous as we were all about nine or ten years old at the time. I climbed trees with the boys, and I played doctors and nurses with them. I would even pretend to lie dead in the road, and they had to come and kiss me back to life. It may explain much of what happened to me later in life.

Next we moved to Bromley and I went to Aylesbury Girls School, and I hated it with a passion. Where were the boys?

They also used to take us on outings. For reasons that I never understood, one of them was to Hampton Court. I wasn't interested. Not one little bit. I preferred to wander around the nearby fields and while I was doing this, I met a boy that I suppose you would describe as the village idiot. We ended up sitting on a bench sharing my sandwiches while he tried to sexually molest me. His hands were everywhere.

He didn't actually know that what he was doing was wrong because he had not been dealt a full pack of cards. In the end, I felt sorry for him and we ended up having a kiss and a fumble in the gardens. I eventually found my way back to the rest of the group, thinking that nobody would have missed me. I couldn't have been more wrong. They had come within a whisker of phoning the police to report me missing. To say that I received a severe reprimand is the understatement of all time.

My hair was all over the place, my tie was undone and I had grass sticking out of my shirt. I looked like something out of St Trinians. Thank goodness they didn't know what the hell I had been up to. And nobody seemed to be too keen to find out.

I didn't care. I just climbed on the coach and headed back to school with a smile on my face. And when they asked us to write about our day at Hampton Court, I came up with some old cobblers about getting lost in the maze and meeting a mad person. The teacher who marked it told me that I would never amount to anything. Some might say she was right, but I will leave you to make your own judgement.

"Sarah, you tell too many lies. You live in a world of your own and you are a Walter Mitty character."

"Whatever, Miss."

My first proper sexual experience was with a girl. Her Mum worked so we would go back to her house after school and experiment. I admit that I fancied her, and it was also me who instigated things. We did things to each other with spoons that are probably best left to the imagination, but let's just say that the two of us experienced a nice warm feeling inside! We also used to throw water over each other – don't ask me why.

I was 11 or 12 years old when this was going on, but I already had a very active sexual imagination. I can vividly remember looking at workmen and wondering if they were well hung. Now you can correct me if I am wrong, but I am fairly certain that not many 12-year-old girls do that – and I haven't the foggiest idea where it came from. But it just all seemed entirely natural. No wonder I failed so miserably at school.

One day I was given detention, which meant that I couldn't catch the bus to my friend's house, and I was really agitated because we had agreed to do our thing with the spoons and I had been looking forward to it.

I caught a later bus and realised I knew the driver. His name was Graham, and he had clearly never looked at me as anything other than a schoolgirl. I hadn't seen this guy for a while and I was sitting talking to him and he realised that something was troubling me.

"What's the matter, Sarah?"

"I've been in detention at school and it means I am too late to go round to my lesbian friend's house and do the spooning thing."

His eyes were like plates and I briefly worried that he was going to crash the bus. I had always been like that though – if people ask me a question, I give them the answer.

Graham was also responsible for my first orgasm, although he didn't know it. I was sitting above one of the wheels on the bus and there was an incredible amount of vibration going on. I got this damp feeling between my legs, not unlike the one I experienced with the spoons, but this was far more powerful. Far, far more powerful.

I remember Graham calling out that he was coming up to my stop. "Fuck that," I thought. "I am going nowhere." And I didn't go anywhere until I'd had the most amazing orgasm. You always remember your first one – and my first one meant that I missed my bloody bus stop.

Most girls have childhood memories that revolve around dolls, but mine are mainly sexual. I had a number of experiences with boys that frustrated me because, well, nothing happened. I am talking about the sort of thing where afterwards you think: "Is that it? Is that all there is?"

I wanted orgasms, like the one I had experienced on the bus.

We never talked about sex in our house. Never. It was a subject that was taboo, out of bounds. Sure, there were the moans and groans that we heard from the bedroom, but that was it. I was a curious child and the only way to satisfy that curiosity was to experiment, to try things out. And I was never afraid to do that.

Mum and Dad would have been horrified if they knew a fraction of what I got up to.

CHAPTER THREE
The Love Of My Life

When I was 14 years old I went on holiday to Devon with my brother and parents. It turned out to be a holiday that would change my life forever because I met a boy called Tony Burge, who was also on holiday with his parents.

Every night in the hotel where we were staying they would have some form of entertainment, and Tony kept staring at me from across the dance floor, and I kept staring back at him. Eventually he came over – it had reached the point where if he hadn't come over and asked me to dance, I was going to ask him.

Our first dance was to the song *Je t'Aime*, which talks about love at first sight. And it was. I was instantly attracted to him. By this point I was attending stage school and although I wasn't used to dancing with boys in the traditional way, like this, I had spent a lot of time dancing with them in the theatrical way, and I really enjoyed it. But not as much as this.

We were inseparable for the entire holiday. He managed to feed me Pernod and blackcurrant and I seemed to spend most of my time happily drunk, having great laughs with this fantastic boy. I didn't see my parents for the entire time we were in Devon, other than at breakfast time.

Our hotel had its own private beach too, so we used to go down there on our own, or have a wander and find deserted coves. It was as if we were the last people alive on earth. And I was as happy as I had ever been in my life. We used to get up to all sorts, and I even ended up back in his bedroom.

Of course the inevitable happened during that holiday and I lost my virginity to Tony, but at least I had waited for the right man to come along! I wasn't to know it at the time, but life held a great deal more in store for Tony and I, individually and as a couple.

Eventually the holiday came to an end and I cried and cried. I couldn't bear to be parted from him. My brother fed off it all the way home, but this was my first love and I was utterly inconsolable.

Tony and his parents lived in Hertfordshire, which was a fair distance from Bromley. They say that love will always find a way, and for about a year it did. We would meet up in London and stay in the cheapest, sleaziest hotels you can imagine. But it didn't matter. I lived for those days when we were together. When I was with Tony, everything was good in my life. All my troubles disappeared.

Sometimes we would also go out with Tony's dad, Ted. He used to say to Tony: "This is a lovely girl. You should look after her and consider yourself lucky to have found such a nice girl." If only he had known. I am sure that I must have been a nice girl once.

"People talk about trophy wives Tony, well Sarah would be amazing by your side, somebody to be proud of, somebody you would be happy to show off." Tony just used to smile because he knew what a sex-mad girl I was.

Ted even used to take us to Institute of Directors' dinners. We had an amazing time.

I should perhaps also explain that not all of our meetings took place at the weekend. There were times when I was so desperate to see him that I would bunk off school and he would do the same. I would head to King's Cross Station, where I would dive into the women's toilet as a 14-

year-old, get changed, apply the slap and emerge as a young woman. Nobody who saw us would have guessed that we were playing truant. We could get into any club, bar or hotel we wanted.

Tony was resourceful, and he always had money. He would wash cars, buy and sell things, whatever it took to put a few bob in his pocket. I knew he would succeed in life, that he would always come up smelling of roses. I suppose you would describe him as a bit of a wide boy.

There was one weekend when his parents were away and I told Dad that I was going to be staying with Tony.

"Are you sure his parents are going to be there?"

"Of course they are Dad. What sort of a daughter do you think you have?"

You should never underestimate your parents. I don't know how, but my father knew that Tony's parents weren't at home and he drove up and dragged me out of a disco. I was screaming and shouting, and Tony was threatening my Dad. He was just doing what any concerned parent would do, and he threw me in the car.

I called him every name under the sun on the way home. I am guessing he was worried that Tony and I were planning to have sex but clearly that particular horse had already bolted. Sorry Dad.

In those days there were no mobile phones, so the only way of keeping in touch with one another was through the house phone, and if he wasn't home when I called then we didn't speak. But it reached the point where he was hardly ever in when I phoned, and Ted would make all sorts of excuses for him.

I began to suspect that he was actually at home but that he simply didn't want to talk to me, and then I thought that he must be seeing somebody else.

One day I decided to catch a train to Welwyn, where he lived, and surprise him. Little did I know that I was the one who was going to be in for the big surprise. So I bought myself a platform ticket and travelled all the way on it. I got off the train and was on my way to catch the bus to his house when I saw him in a record shop. As I started walking towards the shop I suddenly realised that he was with a girl. He hadn't seen me, so I marched into the shop and asked him what was going on.

The girl said: "Who the hell are you?"

I said: "Who the hell are you?"

Tony's face turned red. This was the last thing on earth he had expected, or wanted.

"Calm down, Sarah, let me walk you back to the station."

"You must think I'm stupid. You just want to get rid of me to be with that tart. Is it because she's got blonde hair? [I was brunette at the time] Or is it because she's got bigger tits than me?"

We had a blazing row, during which he told me that I was the last person on earth he would ever marry because I was a raving lunatic. I ended up falling to my knees, begging him not to leave me. This was in the middle of Welwyn Garden City railway station, with hundreds of onlookers unable to believe their eyes.

I was besotted with this boy, but all that he wanted to do was to pack me on a train heading out of his life. He would later tell me that he couldn't cope with the way I flirted with his friends, but he couldn't seem to get it into his head that he was the only one who mattered to me, he was the one I was going home with. It is just the way I am.

Even now, I get accused of making a pass at people when, as far as I am concerned, all that I am doing is having a normal conversation.

That wasn't the end of the story. About six weeks after we split up I discovered that I was pregnant. I told a friend and she insisted that I had to phone Tony and let him know. So I dragged this poor girl along to the phone box with me, rang his number and, for once, it was Tony who answered.

"Oh, what do you want?"

"Tony, I'm pregnant."

"You're lying. You're just saying that." With that, he put down the phone on me.

He was convinced that I was spinning him a line to convince him to take me back. Now I had no choice but to own up to my parents, and you can imagine the scene that followed.

There was a huge shouting match and lots of things were said that we later regretted.

My mother was in denial. "Are you sure? You can't be. How can you be pregnant? No, you can't be. You've made a mistake."

Dad was apoplectic. He went into his pocket and started throwing money at me. "Just get rid of it. Go and get rid of it." This was his way of telling me to go and have an abortion. I look back on it now and smile, but that was the way people dealt with things back then.

And then he wanted to know who the father was. The baby was Tony's, but despite the way he had treated me, I didn't want my Dad turning up on his doorstep, so I said: "Well it could be one of several boys."

So rather than pointing the finger at Tony, who had been an utter bastard to me, I gave my Dad the impression that I was some sort of teenage slag who was sleeping with half the population. In the end I went to see my doctor, who referred me to a clinic which performed the abortion. My mother wouldn't even go with me, telling me to phone her when it was over.

I duly picked up the phone and told her the abortion had been performed and there was a brief silence on the other end before she put the phone down. The subject was never brought up again.

And Tony disappeared from my life. But he would reappear...

CHAPTER FOUR
Reaching For The Stars

I took elocution lessons at my mother's insistence, and my teacher saw something in me that nobody else had, and suggested that I audition for a stage school.

"You are a very talented girl Sarah, and you should be finding a way to make the most of it. I think you would blossom at stage school, and you would love the experience." Remember that up until this point, I'd had to put up with teachers telling me that I wouldn't amount to anything, so this came as a huge confidence booster.

I was an outgoing child. I loved to perform for people, and I enjoyed being the centre of attention. My idol was Bette Davis, the Hollywood actress. Although she may not have been a beauty in the traditional sense, she possessed something special.

And yes, I enjoyed being on stage. Getting up and performing to an audience – wow! Have you any idea what a powerful thing it is to be up there acting a part or singing a song, knowing that everybody is watching you? And the feeling when you have finished and you hear the applause. For a young teenage girl it was something special, and I quickly became addicted. I never saw it as acting – I was just being me.

At the age of 12, I auditioned for the Italia Conti stage school in London. I had to dance, act and sing and, lo and behold, I was accepted. I have no recollection of the song I sang or of the lines that I read, but I do remember that I performed a tap-dancing routine. I loved tap-dancing with a passion and took part in lots of shows in and around

Bromley when I was growing up.

My parents were thrilled when I was accepted. It meant that they had to pay fees but they felt it was an opportunity that wasn't offered to many kids and they were determined that I was going to make the most of it.

The school was exactly as you would expect – a combination of traditional lessons with acting, singing and dance classes. You can imagine, too, how incredibly precocious most of my fellow students were. It was full of luvvies, and it wasn't terribly strict. And that suited me down to the ground.

You will have heard of some of my fellow pupils – Tracey Ullman, Leslie Ash, David Van Day, Peter Duncan, Patsy Kensitt. There were also many, many more you will never have heard of, boys and girls who failed to make it and were later forced to take "proper" jobs. There was also a boy called Paul Gadd, whose father was Gary Glitter – whenever Glitter turned up at the school, it seemed to me that he always wanted to get up on stage and perform. And he was always happy to help out in the changing rooms – knowing what I know now about him, the mind boggles. But back then he was one of the most famous pop stars on the planet.

I excelled at elocution, perhaps because I'd already had lessons. Unbelievably, I was the teacher's pet. This sort of thing didn't happen to me. The teacher was a big stern woman who used to whack a stick on the floor and make you jump six feet in the air if you got anything wrong, but I never got anything wrong.

I used to be able to do all sorts of accents, although I can't do it anymore.

A typical day would consist of perhaps academic classes in the morning, say maths, English and geography, and then you would have your lunch and in the afternoon it would be one of the three main theatrical disciplines (acting, singing and dance). There always seemed to be rehearsals going on for something or other because the school put on its own shows, as well as sending pupils out to auditions for all sorts of shows.

I made a good friend called Wendy Hornby, and I also got to know the late Lena Zavaroni, who arrived after winning *Opportunity Knocks*. Although she was younger than me, Lena became a close friend. She was as thin as a rake and very quiet when she wasn't performing. A lot of the kids were like that – they would be fairly shy until they got into character, and then it was as if they had put on some sort of mask. Suddenly they would come to life.

I thought it was a shame that it took a song or lines that had been written by somebody else to switch on a person. It would have been so much better had they been able to relate to people as themselves, rather than as the characters they became.

I kept bumping into Patsy Kensitt at auditions. She had originally attended a different stage school before moving to Italia Conti, and I got sick of the sight of her. Patsy was a brilliant young actress, and if I saw her at an audition I knew that I was wasting my time being there because she would almost always get the part.

"Okay, thanks girls. We will let you know." Yeah, right! After you, Patsy.

My biggest claim to fame while I was at Italia Conti came when they were casting *Jesus of Nazareth*, starring Robert Powell, and they were looking for somebody to play the young Virgin Mary. Stop laughing at the back!

This was the big time, a Franco Zeffirelli production. The way it works is that when a play, film or whatever is due to be made, notices will be sent to schools such as the Italia Conti, telling them what parts are available and the type of young actor or actress the director is looking for.

Franco wanted three people to play the Virgin Mary at various stages of her life – a young child, somebody to play her aged 12-16 and a mature actress to play her as an adult. I was told that I should apply for the part and I duly went along to the audition process, which was one of the most gruelling things I have ever done.

There were hundreds of girls up for the part, and I do mean hundreds. And they had to see each and every one of them. I always struggled to get myself noticed at Italia Conti – not among the teachers, many of whom thought I possessed a fair amount of talent, but among my peers. We would sit down and discuss who should be cast for this part or that role, and it seemed that my name never came up.

But this was different. As the potential Virgins were being whittled down, they kept asking me back. I thought there must be some mistake, but it finally registered with me that I had a realistic chance of being offered this role.

In the end, there were five of us left standing and we all had to audition in person for Zeffirelli. I don't mind telling you that it was a pretty terrifying ordeal because although I didn't really know who this man was, I was cute enough to realise that he was somebody pretty important. Anyway, I must have done something right because I was told that I was being given the part. Because I looked so angelic apparently! And because I spoke so well. Mum was right about those elocution lessons after all.

They announced in assembly that I had been successful and had been chosen to play the Virgin Mary, aged 12 to 16, and every body stood up and applauded me. What a feeling that was. I was ecstatic. All the hard work had paid off.

"I've done it! My God, I've done it!"

Some of my fellow pupils were less than enthusiastic with their praise. I could see it in their eyes. They were thinking: "How the hell has she got the part?"

I have to say that two of the worst were Leslie Ash and Tracey Ullman. They were fine until you landed a part that they wanted, and then they were absolutely horrible to me and took the piss. After I got the part of the Virgin Mary, all the petty jealousies came to the fore, and I endured a fairly miserable time. Why couldn't they just have been happy for me? As it turned out, they didn't do so badly for themselves, did they? And I was never going to steal their thunder anyway because it was perfectly clear that they were far more talented than I ever was.

But this was my moment, and I wanted to enjoy it. Fat chance. I would walk past and hear comments being made about the way I looked or the fact that I was too skinny. It was hurtful. It was as if they wanted to extract any feelings of pleasure I had experienced, like they wanted to drag me down and destroy my confidence before I had even started filming. How cruel was that?

It made me want to go away and slit my wrists. There were enough issues among the pupils without this. When she first arrived at the school, Lena Zavaroni was actually quite a chubby little girl, but before long she was becoming as image conscious as the rest of us. She started off by skipping the odd meal, and the weight fell off her. The problem was that, in the process, she had become anorexic, and she wasn't the only one. I am sure that those who became anorexic used to look at themselves in the mirror and convince themselves that if they were a little bit thinner they would have a better chance of getting the part they wanted. It starts with skipping the odd meal, but before long it becomes a full-blown illness. Even back then, image was everything.

The last thing that these individuals need is to have people chipping away at their confidence. I was never going to do anything stupid, but I simply couldn't understand why they couldn't just be pleased for me. When all was said and done, a pupil from the Italia Conti School was about to star in possibly the biggest television production of all time.

Unsurprisingly, I began to feel totally stressed out, and before I knew where I was, my face was covered in spots. Thankfully, I decided against resorting to a cure I had tried once before during my time at Italia Conti – I figured that if I dabbed bleach onto cotton wool and then onto my face that it would not only get rids of spots but it might even prevent them from coming back. I couldn't understand why nobody had tried it before. I soon realised why! It got rid of the spots all right, but when I woke up my face was stinging. I looked in the mirror and screamed – the bleach had effectively burnt my skin.

Rather than owning up to what I had done, I sneaked downstairs with a hot-water bottle, filled it up with boiling hot water, waited until it cooled down and then pretended it had burst open on my face. What a scheming bitch I was, even back then. My mother took me to the doctor and of course I couldn't tell him the truth either so he just had a quick look and announced that it would be all right. Jesus! I was suffering from the equivalent of third-degree burns.

As the weeks passed, so my skin started to peel and eventually it healed, but I learnt a lesson. The funny thing is that I later realised that I was ahead of my time and that I had probably invented the first facial peel! I was so lucky that I did not permanently scar myself but the bottom line is that I did it because of the pressure I felt I was always under to look my best at Italia Conti, and because I knew that I probably didn't possess the natural looks of some of my classmates, I took matters into my own hands. I look back now and shudder at what I might have done to my looks although, as it turned out, somebody else would end up doing the most unspeakable things to my face.

So yes, I was stressed out again, even though I had landed this amazing part, but I was also as high as a kite. At this stage I believed that I was going to be playing a part in a movie. Contracts were flying backwards and forwards and I was being told that I couldn't do this, but I had to do that. I was given the dates when they wanted me to be at the studio. Suddenly, my life was being controlled by faceless men and women I had never met, but I was told that I had to toe the line, and I duly did as I was told. Why would I want to rock the boat?

Everything was going great. Right up until the point where they ran out of money and announced that the project was being shelved. I was devastated.

Of course, Zeffirelli managed to get the project refinanced, but this time as a mammoth TV series, and he went and cast Olivia Hussey as the Virgin Mary. Can you imagine how I felt as I heard what was happening? I had done nothing wrong. Nothing. It wasn't my fault that there wasn't enough money in the pot, but I was the one who was cast aside. It made me want to chuck the whole thing in. I have nothing against Olivia, who was fantastic in the part? She also had the kind of face that meant she could get away with playing the Virgin Mary from the age of 12 right through to adulthood, which meant they could keep costs down. Could I have done it as well as her? We will never know.

And if I had starred in the television series, would my life have played out any differently? It might well have done.

So I had to try and pick myself up and get on with it, but I really didn't feel inclined to do so. Going along to an audition and not getting the part is something you learn to deal with – budding actors and actresses get rejected far more often than they are successful. In fact, if truth be told, precisely the same thing applies to actors and actresses who have established themselves. The whole audition process can be soul destroying and if you don't have thick skin (whether it has been treated with bleach or not), then you really should be looking for an alternative profession.

But this wasn't like that. I had done everything that had been asked of me. I had worked my socks off and gone back to audition after audition, often when I felt like telling them what they could do with themselves. I was young and I suppose that I was ambitious – at the very least, somebody should have sat me down, put an arm around me and explained what had happened. Instead, I was left to pick up the pieces on my own.

To come so close and have it grabbed away really hurt. Needless to say, many of my fellow students took great delight in my plight.

This all happened at about the time that I had fallen pregnant with Tony's baby and it was just about the final straw. I suppose that I lost interest. I am a competitive person and I don't like finishing second in anything. My solution was to start bunking off, and nobody seemed to care too much.

I was never taken to task for failing to turn up at lessons, so maybe the teachers had given up on me as well.

CHAPTER FIVE
Awakenings ...

So what does a teenage girl with no interest in school do with her herself to pass the time when she is playing truant? I suppose that most normal girls would have spent the time at a friend's house, or maybe in a park. Perhaps they would wander round the shops.

I was never your typical teenage girl though, and I decided to hang out at Victoria train station. I haven't a clue why, but it ended up changing my life forever.

I didn't want to tell my parents that I was fed up with Italia Conti and no longer wanted to go there because I knew that they had invested a lot of time and money in it on my behalf. I would have been better off coming clean and admitting that it wasn't for me, but that would have been too easy. And I also knew that I didn't want to return to mainstream schooling. That would have been awful.

So I would leave home in the morning and as far as Mum and Dad were concerned, I was going to Italia Conti. And sometimes I did even go to the school. On other occasions I would take entire days off, or I would go in for registration and then clear off. I would even forge letters, saying that I had a dental appointment, or a hospital appointment.

The strange thing is that I was still getting auditions, which means that somebody at the school believed in me. I even auditioned for *The Benny Hill Show*, but although I had the legs, at that time I was flat-chested and I was never going to be offered a part as one of his so-called Angels. I knew my shortcomings and remember telling Hill that I could stuff my bra if it would help. He was a really sweet man and said: "That's great Sarah, but the thing is that you are not quite right. Not yet anyway." He offered me some kind of hope that maybe if I came back a few months later then there might be something for me.

Stuff that for a game of soldiers.

I also auditioned for Legs And Co, the dancers who used to appear on *Top Of The Pops*, but I kept getting to the brink and they kept saying: "Thanks but no thanks." I was either too short, too tall, too skinny, too flat-chested. There was always something.

The most frustrating thing of all was that I kept getting called back after first auditions, and that raised my hopes because I kept thinking: "Perhaps this is the one. This is where they say that they want me, where they tell me that I am exactly what they are looking for." And then I would get the letter or the phone call. More often than not, I didn't even get that. It is a shabby way to treat human beings who are chasing their dreams, and it is no wonder that so many fall by the wayside.

It doesn't matter how it is dressed up - rejection is a horrible thing.

So let's stop for a moment to examine where I was in my life. I'd been dumped by my boyfriend, I'd had an abortion, my relationship with my parents was not in a good place, I had been kicked in the guts after being led to believe that I had landed a dream role, and I was being singled out and picked on by my fellow students. I was not in a good place.

And I wasn't the only one. I looked around me, especially at the girls, and most of them seemed to be developing anxieties. It is hardly surprising when you think about it. In what other environment would you put a child through a situation where they spend most of their lives being told that they are not right for a part, that their singing voice isn't quite what the director had in mind, that they are too fat, too thin. It is hard to take at any age, but it is surely most difficult when you are growing up, trying to do the thing you want to do more than anything else in the world.

Some of the kids stopped eating and developed conditions such as anorexia, while others went the opposite way and started comfort eating. And then you would see children's personalities changing as they became ever more introverted and withdrawn. Not everybody was like this, of course – some of the kids positively thrived in the environment, but they were in the minority.

I watched beautiful girls fall apart as they developed insecurities about the way they looked. It wasn't pleasant.

I knew from almost the first time that I met her that Ullman was going to make it. She was fabulous at everything she turned her hand to, but she was not a pleasant individual, well not to me at any rate. It struck me that she went out of her way to make certain people very unhappy, and I could never understand why. It costs nothing to be nice. She was and is a great mimic and she used to ape teachers and pupils. Sometimes it was funny, but just as often it was cruel.

I am sure that she is a very different person now, although I do understand that to become as successful as she has, perhaps you need to possess a ruthless streak.

Leslie Ash was another who possessed star quality at an early age. She was blonde and beautiful, even when she was snivelling away with a cold. There was something special about her. She had an aura and all the boys fancied the pants off her.

Peter Duncan, the former *Blue Peter* presenter, attended Italia Conti, as did his sister, Julia Gayle, and I got to know Julia quite well. There must be a reason why they had different surnames, but I am not sure what it was. Anyway, the family had a home not far from Bromley and their parents must have been away because Peter organised a weekend party, and all the invitations went out.

I was asked, not because I was part of Peter's inner sanctum, but because I lived nearby. Dad said that I could go but first of all he went round to see Peter and explained to him that I was only 14 years old. "I am allowing my daughter to stay overnight at your place, but you have to promise that you will look after her and make sure that nothing happens to her." Peter, by the way, was at least four years older than me and the last thing on earth he would have wanted to do was to babysit me, but he duly gave Dad the necessary assurances.

Within minutes of arriving at the house on the Saturday night, it became clear that everything was out of control, with dozens upon dozens of gatecrashers arriving. It was carnage. There were bikers. There were people having sex on the front lawn. The drink flowed and before long people were throwing up, and I am certain that there were also drugs being handed around. People were smoking cigarettes and stubbing them out on the carpets.

I remember lying on the sofa at one point, pissed as a fart, allowing two boys to grope me. I was so far gone that they could have done anything they wanted to me and I wouldn't have been able to do anything about it. In the end, we all finished up in bed and had a good old shag. Poor old Dad would have had a fit.

I remember looking around at one point and it seemed that just about everybody was naked. And then, inevitably, fights began to break out. It was utter chaos.

Afterwards, the house was completely wrecked, but when everybody woke up on the Sunday morning nobody seemed to care. We carried on partying until all the booze was gone and then cleared off before Peter's parents came home. We left him to face the music.

I got home and Dad asked: "Did you have a good time Sarah?"

"Yes Dad, not bad. It was a quiet night, but it was all right."

I wasn't quite finished with Italia Conti yet. One of the few lessons I did attend was maths, because I developed a crush on Mr Anderson, the teacher. Just like Tony, he also had red hair.

I was never any good at mathematics, and because I was so bad he used to keep me behind. "We are going to go over this again and again until you understand it Sarah, no matter how many times it takes. This is important. You've got exams coming up."

I would undo a couple of buttons on my blouse or pull my skirt up too high, just to see what sort of reaction I could get from him. He always pretended not to notice, but he knew precisely what I was up to. I was bored, and I wanted to have a bit of fun. Needless to say, although I wanted him to have his evil way with me, he always behaved impeccably. Bastard!

I never did learn anything though.

Eventually it reached the point where I was spending just about all day, every day at Victoria Station reading books, waiting for the appointed hour to jump on a train back home.

"Good day at school Sarah?"

"Yes thanks Mum."

There was a coffee bar at Victoria station, and I used to sit there and make a cup of coffee last for hours. Eventually, I was approached by a man who had spent weeks watching me, waiting to make his move.

He was a Scot and he introduced himself to me as Jock. Very original. But it didn't register with me. He asked me what I was reading and I told him, and then he asked why I was wearing a school uniform.

"I am bunking off school."

"Your parents obviously don't know."

"Of course they don't, and they never will."

I had never met this man before in my life, and here I was blurting it all out, and loud enough so that everybody else in the cafe could hear me too. I even told him that I forged notes, got the train at a specific time, and I also informed him where I lived. It was incredibly naive, but although I pretended to be streetwise, I really wasn't.

"What school do you go to?"

"The Italia Conti theatre school."

"Why don't you want to go there then? I would have thought that would be great fun."

He was digging away, trying to get as much information as he could from me, and there I was feeding it all to him without so much as a second thought. I knew nothing about this man, other than the fact that he was called Jock and he lived in Denbigh Street, round the back of the station.

"Let me buy you a drink. You've been here for a few days and you have been really engrossed in that book."

So now I knew that he had been eyeing me for sometime, although I had never noticed him before, and he was happy for me to know that; in fact, he had gone out of way to let me know. I should have been worried, but I wasn't. I don't know why, but I felt completely in control of both this man and of the situation.

He was skinny and his hair was greasy. God's gift to women he was not. In truth, he looked like a bit of a pervert, and I suppose that is exactly what he was because he clearly knew that I was under-age and it didn't put him off one little bit. On the contrary. I don't know what age he was, but he was much, much older than me. I would guess he was about 40.

He had a cigarette hanging out the corner of his mouth, and his teeth and fingers were stained by nicotine, and here I was chatting away to him like he was my new best mate. I should have been running a mile in the opposite direction.

The penny should have dropped by now, but it still hadn't. He sat next to me and we chatted, and then it was time for me to go home.

"He seemed nice," I thought to myself. "Perhaps I will meet him again tomorrow."

And sure enough, I went back to Victoria the following day and there he was. Once again, he bought me a coffee and a cake. This went on for days, and then weeks, and all the time I was getting closer to him. I didn't realise it, but the bastard was grooming me. There is no other word for it.

And then the inevitable happened.

"Why are we sitting here Sarah? Why don't we go back to mine? It's only just around the corner. We can have a drink there, it will be more comfortable, and you will not have to worry about anybody recognising you."

"Oh all right then."

"But don't tell your parents because they won't like me. This will just be our little secret."

How stupid was I?

By now, I trusted him totally, even though I still knew nothing about him at all. He had found out everything there was to know about me, but it was all one way.

He put his arm around me and led me to his bedsit. It was revolting and I immediately asked myself: "What the hell am I doing here?"

There was a bed, a cooker and a chair, and that was about it.

Then he asked if I wanted a cup of tea, and suggested it would taste better with a shot of whisky in it. And it did! I sat on the edge of the bed and we chatted and, as we did so, girls kept knocking on his front door.

There were whispered conversations and money and packages were changing hands and although I thought it all seemed a bit odd, I convinced myself that they must all be his friends, and that I was the special one. After all, I was the one he had made the tea for, and I was the one he kept meeting in the station cafe.

I heard one woman say to him: "Who is she? She's wearing a school uniform Jock – what are you doing? Be careful."

"Don't worry about it. I know what I am doing."

Still the penny hadn't dropped. Was I thick, or what?

We got talking again and now I felt confident enough to tell him about Tony, and about my first sexual experiences. I even told him that I had got myself pregnant.

"You could have anyone you want Sarah, you do know that don't you? You are a beautiful girl."

He sat next to me. "Look at all those freckles – I could play dot-to-dot with the freckles on your thigh."

Nothing further happened on that first day, but he agreed to meet me the next day, and I ended up back in his hell-hole of a bedsit again. And this time he asked me if I wanted to earn some money.

"Of course I'd like to make some money. What would I have to do?"

"Certain things."

"What do you mean?"

"With men, in your school uniform. Instead of sitting at Victoria station all day being bored out of your mind, you could make a few quid."

"But what would I have to do?"

"Pleasure men, Sarah."

I hadn't a clue what he was on about and told him so.

"Let me show you..."

And with that, he dropped his trousers, took my hand and taught me how to masturbate him. I should have been shocked, but I can honestly say that I wasn't. Even though I say so myself, I took to it like a duck to water. When I eventually left school, I did not have a single qualification to my name, but I was the best little wanker in town! And it was all down to what Jock showed me.

I should have been repulsed by it all but instead I found myself thinking: "If men are prepared to pay me for doing this then how stupid are they? I will definitely have a piece of that action."

Did it occur to me that he was trying to turn me into a teenage prostitute? An under-age teenage prostitute? An under-age teenage prostitute whose father was a high-flying officer in the Metropolitan police force! Even I realised that you couldn't make this up, and that if you did, nobody would believe you.

"I want to leave school anyway, so I might as well sit here and make some money. Jock's not such a bad chap." I convinced myself it was the right thing to do – a good career move, if you like. Had I lost my marbles?

Naturally, I couldn't go home and tell Mum and Dad about my new career choice, but I informed Jock that I was prepared to give it a go. Let's get one thing straight. Although I didn't want to hurt Jock's feelings by saying no, this was my decision. Nobody forced me. I never did find out what Jock's real name was, although I did get to know him pretty intimately as he taught me everything that I needed to know about sex, and about making a man feel 10 feet tall.

Once he had taught me, he said: "Right Sarah, I can get men to come and visit you here [in the bedsit] and pay you to have sex with them. It will be completely safe for you. I will never be too far away."

And off he would go and scout for punters, so at least he didn't have me hanging around on street corners, and I suppose that I should be grateful for that.

Incredibly, he brought back a string of supposedly respectable men – teachers, judges, and magistrates. And then there were the weirdos who would produce whips and canes from their briefcases – I mean, did these guys walk around all day carrying these things with them, just in case? Some of these guys were sick. When they went off to work for the day, what did they tell their wives?

So here I was, a fully-fledged under-age prostitute. Although I have stressed that nobody forced me to do any of this, Jock groomed me, and he knew exactly what he was doing. He saw an attractive, vulnerable girl who was looking for a bit of excitement, and he exploited me. Worse than that, all the men who paid to have sex with me did so because they wanted to make love to an under-age girl. I don't know quite what that tells you about society, but I promise you there were no shortage of them.

The ones I worried about were the teachers. I hoped that by having their way with me, it was enough to satisfy them, but I will never know. When all is said and done, what they were doing to me amounted to child abuse of the worst possible kind, but they convinced themselves it was all right because they were paying for the privilege.

I make no excuses for myself, although there were times when I was quite staggered at how busy he was. And if he was busy, then so was I. Jock used to wait outside and the men would pay him. I have no idea how much he was charging them, and I haven't a clue how much he pocketed. All that I do know is that he didn't give me very much. But I didn't care.

This went on for about a year and then one morning I woke up, decided I'd had enough and never went back to the bedsit in Denbigh

Street. I suppose that I'd had a moment of enlightenment – if I stayed with Jock, I could see this awful life playing out in front of me. I would probably end up hooked on drugs or drink, or both. There would probably have been another unwanted pregnancy or two. It had been fun while it lasted, but no more, thank you very much.

At around about the same time, I got the results of my exams, and I managed to fail every single subject, which hardly came as a surprise to me. Dad was furious. He seemed to spend a great deal of his life shouting at me. I know that I was a constant disappointment.

There was a time when he hired a private tutor to help me out with maths and English. His name was Mr Woodwark, and I tried to come on to him too. In any event, the tuition was a waste of time and money. I remember him telling my father that I was thick and that he could never get through to me. I wasn't thick – I just hated maths. I was good at sex because I enjoyed it.

CHAPTER SIX
Going Like A Rabbit

My attitude to life has always been that something will turn up, and that was no different after I gave Jock the heave-ho. I knew that something would come along, even though I was stepping out into the big bad world without a single qualification to my name.

I registered with a number of employment agencies but they weren't desperately enthusiastic because as far as they were concerned I did not have a great deal offer. And as far as I was aware, being a great wanker was not a job qualification and was unlikely to open too many doors for me (I would later discover that I could not be more mistaken).

Somebody wanted to turn me into a switchboard operator, but I really didn't fancy that. Apart from anything else, can you imagine the utter mayhem that I would have caused? Nobody would have ended up speaking to the person they expected to be talking to.

My first proper job was as a house model and part-time receptionist at the Alexon Fashion House. A house model is somebody who tries on clothes for buyers. It is not rocket science and it is not challenging, but it helped to pay the bills, and I never regarded it as anything other than a stop-gap, something to fill in the time until a better offer came along. Besides, I used to spend a good deal of my time having sex with the boss, in his office.

At least it was all legal by this time – I was 16 by now.

I stuck it out for a year, during which time I bumped into Tony Burge again. There was still a bit of something between us, but I had been hurt by the way he treated me. He wanted to pick things up again, but I was very wary of him and although I agreed to go for a meal, that was as far as it went. I didn't see him again after that until much, much later in my life.

One day on my way home from work I picked up the *Evening Standard* and I was flicking through job pages when I noticed an advert for the Playboy Club. They were looking for croupiers. Don't forget that I was awful with numbers, but I felt that I had nothing to lose, so I phoned the number in the advert and was given an audition time – it was like being back at Italia Conti.

Mind you, I should have realised that it was never going to be a formal interview. This was the Playboy Club, home of the Bunny Girl, and it was highly unlikely that they would ever be interested in much more than my looks and my ability to string a few words together.

I had to met the Bunny Mother, whose name was Erin Stratton, and she also had a sidekick. I had been told to bring a swimming costume, but I have to admit that I hadn't a clue what the Playboy Club was all about. I realised you probably had to be good-looking to get a job there, and I figured that it was probably patronised by lots of rich and famous people. But that was it. That was the extent of my knowledge.

I didn't know what a Bunny Girl actually did, although I had a vague idea that some of them had their pictures taken for top-shelf magazines.

I had a couple of weeks to get ready for the audition, and spent the whole time worrying about which swimsuit I should wear. I'd been lambasted at Italia Conti for having no hips and no bum, so I created some implants which I stitched into a swimming costume, and suddenly I had a curvaceous bum. By then, my breasts had finally developed so at least I no longer had issues with a flat chest.

I arrived for the audition and was sent into a changing room, but when I put the suit on it just didn't look right, and I ended up spending ages in there pulling and prodding, poking and pushing. In the end, I ripped out the implants.

"Are you all right in there, Sarah?"

"Yes, yes, I'm fine."

"We haven't got all day you know. We have other girls to see."

When I finally emerged, Erin simply said: "Perfect. That's perfect, absolutely perfect."

I figured that I might be in with half a chance when I heard that. As she stood looking at me she was making notes and asking questions, and then came the fateful one.

"How old are you Sarah?"

"I'm 18," I lied.

"Perfect."

Eighteen was the minimum age you had to be. I was 17, and if I had owned up to that I would have been shown the door without any hesitation, and I wasn't prepared to lose this opportunity.

They had to decide whether I would be best as a croupier bunny or as a straightforward waitress bunny, so I was given a simple maths test. Needless to say, I failed it quite spectacularly. That was that, then. If I was going to be working here, it was going to be as a waitress.

I was shown around the club. It was pretty dark and dingy, with images of racehorses on the walls. I was then told: "We will let you know." I'd heard that line often enough to walk away expecting never to hear from them again. But the next thing I knew was that I was being asked when I could start. I was ecstatic, absolutely ecstatic.

I then had to undergo an induction and quickly realised that I had to learn the precise ingredients of every cocktail known to man – and some that weren't. Perhaps this was going to be a bit more difficult than I had imagined.

The way it worked was that if you were doing a day shift there would be fewer staff working, so I would take the order and then have to make the drinks myself and bring them back for the customers. At night, when it was busy, you just handed the order over to the barman. There were some weird and wonderful concoctions, I can tell you. A Slow Screw On The Beach While The Tide Is Coming In, a White Angel With Devil In Her Hair, a Fast Screw Up Against The Side Of Washing Machine....okay, so I am exaggerating, but not by much.

There was a manual and it was at least an inch thick, that listed every possible combination. When a customer asked for a drink, it would never do to ask what was in it. You had to nod your head wisely, pretend you knew precisely what he or she wanted and then dive to the bar, thumb through the manual and hope it was listed. This manual also listed all the rules and regulations – it told us how to open a bottle of champagne, it told us how to perform what was known as the 'bunny dip' correctly. And it told us what we could and what we could not say to the customers. Essentially, we were not meant to speak until we were spoken to – as you can imagine, I found that something of a challenge.

A job that I thought was going to be a piece of cake turned out to be rather more difficult that I had ever imagined it could be. I realised the only way I could master it all was to go back to the days when I would learn a script parrot fashion – and that is precisely what I did. It took a while, and I made a few screw-ups along the way, but suddenly it just all seemed to click. I knew the entire contents of the manual, backwards, forwards, sideways.

And best of all, for the first time in my life I was earning proper money. Most of the punters were Arabs and they would throw money at you, money which I would stuff down the front of my costume. You would then go to the bar, pay for the drinks and keep the rest. I felt 10 feet tall. I knew that there was no way that I would have been given this job unless the Bunny Mother had thought I looked the part, and knowing that just made me, and all the other girls, feel special.

I was turning into a beautiful young woman, and I knew it. A beautiful young woman who had done some very, very naughty things but, hey, we all have to grow up, don't we? We all have to make our mistakes and learn from them? The thing is that nobody else I knew had made their mistakes pleasuring seedy, perverted men in a grotty bedsit round the corner from Victoria Station. Thank God those days were behind me.

All that I had to do was serve drinks to these men and smile. I would come home after a shift, take off my bunny costume and hundreds of pounds would fall on the floor, thousands of pounds sometimes. The Arabs would also hand over gambling chips and I would cash those in at the end of the night – and the minimum chip you would receive would be £100.

Of course they gave us the money because they wanted to go out with us. And they wanted to go out with us so that they could take us back to a flat or a hotel and make love to us. Nothing was for nothing. One of the chief house rules was that we were not allowed to fraternise with the punters, but do you think that anybody paid attention to that? Of course they didn't.

Besides, the management knew what was going on. Everybody was at it with everybody else. It was a glorified knocking shop full of beautiful young women who virtually prostituted themselves. In that sense, nothing had changed for me. Except that it couldn't have been more different. These men were incredibly wealthy and, in the main, they treated us like royalty, and were prepared to pay whatever it took to get what they wanted.

We went out with these men, they lavished us with gifts, but we knew precisely why they were spending all this money on us. Dress it up any way you choose, but they wanted just one thing from us. Almost all of them had wives tucked away, so we knew that we were never going to be given any sort of commitment. This was sex, pure and simple. Well, not so pure actually, and not always so simple.

Victor Lownes ran the Park Lane club where I worked, and Hugh Hefner, the head honcho, would visit from time to time. I hadn't a clue who he was either, or what he stood for, but whenever he would appear everybody seemed to be extra nervous. It was like we had visiting royalty on the premises. I was never one to stand on ceremony though. My attitude was, and still is, that people have to take me as they find me.

My first encounter with Hefner was one I will never forget. He walked into the club and was shown to a table and lots of people were fussing about him when I was told: "Right then Sarah, you are the new girl, and Hef always likes to check out the new girls, so you go and serve him. And don't fuck it up."

I marched up to the table and there he was, in the company of a beautiful young girl who had the worst fake tan I have ever seen. As I looked down I saw a giant cockroach on his table so I smashed it with my hand, killing it on the white tablecloth. I didn't even blink. It just seemed the natural thing to do. Here was the owner of the Playboy empire sitting at one of my tables and there was a bloody cockroach. What was I supposed to do? Ignore it? Hope it would go away?

I didn't think I had done anything wrong, but I suddenly became aware that everybody was frozen to the spot and I could feel all these eyes on me. Nobody said a word. I looked at Hefner and hoped that he might crack a smile, but there was nothing. People were looking at

Hefner waiting for him to react, and I could hear someone throwing a fit. It was only a bloody cockroach, for God's sake!

You must have seen those old Westerns where a stranger comes into town, walks into the bar and everything stops, apart from maybe a piece of tumbleweed blowing down the street. That is exactly what it was like.

Then I heard somebody say: "Get that girl off the floor now! Hugh is going to blow up any minute."

Eventually Hefner spoke. "Come upstairs with me. I need to talk to you in private."

Naturally, I followed. I was sure he was going to fire me, but he led me to an office and as soon as we got inside he turned to face me and started taking off his trousers and instructed me to give him a blow job, but he actually came before I could. Then he got cross and I said: "I have always been good at that."

By now, I'd got this daft idea that perhaps he was going to offer me a job in America, but I soon realised that wasn't the case at all. Mind you, I did have something on him – he would not have wanted anybody to know what I had just seen, that the guy had come all over his pants without me laying a finger on him.

It all ended with him saying something like: "Okay, that'll do. Go back to your work." And he gave me a look that left me in no doubt that it would not be a good idea to say anything to my colleagues.

When I returned to the bar, the barman gave me a knowing look: "I bet you got a right telling off."

"Not half."

I went back to work but was totally flustered and kept getting orders wrong and tripping over things. My nerves were shot to pieces, and I suddenly felt that everybody was watching my every move. It was horrible.

And eventually I heard Hefner screaming: "Get that woman out of my sight right now."

That was my first encounter with the man, and by far the most memorable. He would turn up on a regular basis, but I never had that sort of contact with him again. Thank goodness.

I didn't like Victor Lownes one little bit. He could never keep his hands off the girls, and he was also a nasty piece of work. He thought that he was God's gift to women, and he had an insatiable appetite for sex. Stories used to go round the club about him having upwards of five women a day, and he would frequently have two at a time.

They used to have parties in the country at a mansion owned by Lownes. The mansion had lots and lots of bedrooms, inside which celebrities and rich Arabs would make love to the chosen few Bunny Girls. This was a glorified knocking shop and even way back then when I heard what was going on I thought that there was money to be made from staging sex parties. If you could provide the beautiful women and some discreet surroundings, then you were on to a winner.

I was never asked, but I always kept my ear close to the ground to find out what was going on. I was more interested in the seedier side of things than I was in doing my job. I used to see money changing hands, and packets and packages would be passed over and under tables, obviously containing drugs. I saw briefcases being swapped, where you would see somebody walking out with a case that he hadn't walked in with.

I was meeting rich Arabs in the club and in a coffee shop on Park Lane. You would be invited to Spain at the drop of a hat. "Come with me and join me on my yacht for two weeks. We will have a great time – you will have a great time." The invitations came thick and fast, but none of us could take them up because if we had, it would have meant losing our jobs.

In many ways I remained quite naive, but I wasn't entirely stupid. The Playboy Club was giving me a regular income; if I went off with a rich Arab, it would be fine until he grew tired of me and dumped me for a newer model. What would I do then? I knew that I had to look after number one.

Don't get me wrong – there were long weekends and the occasional holiday spent on yachts, and I was taken shopping in stores such as Harrods and Harvey Nicholls. These men knew how to treat a woman, or perhaps I should say that they knew what they had to do in order to get what they wanted.

Diamonds, fur coats, designer watches, gold rings – the amount of money that was lavished on me and my fellow employees was mind-boggling, but it was petty cash to these men. It was obscene.

By and large, the Arabs treated us superbly when they wanted us around, but then they would decide that they wanted to do a bit of business and I would be dismissed, expected to make myself scarce until I was needed again. So in many respects I felt like a possession. Put it this way – I knew where I stood in the grand scheme of things, so I decided to enjoy the best bits and milk it for everything I possibly could. If a man wanted to spend thousands of pounds on me, who was I to stop him?

"I am busy now Sarah. Here's some money – go shopping." There were worse ways to live, and there were worse ways to be treated. And don't forget – I was still only 17 years old.

My other abiding memory of those days concerns the vast amounts of cocaine these men would use – industrial amounts of the stuff. They didn't care what it cost, and there would be lots of it scattered over glass tables. I dread to think how much was simply swept off the tables, onto the floor and, ultimately, into the bowels of a vacuum cleaner.

I was never interested in cocaine, or any other drug. I dabbled with marijuana when I was about 11 years old but I didn't enjoy it, and of course I tried the cocaine during my Bunny Girl days but it made me go wild and I knew that it wasn't good news, so I stopped. As a young girl, I also had my father coming home and telling us awful stories about people he had arrested, and what their drug addiction had done to them. I knew how addictive cocaine could be, so figured that the best thing was just to leave well alone, and that's what I did. I suppose that I had to sample it just to get an idea and a feeling for what everybody around me was getting from it.

With the sort of personality I have, I would have wanted more and more and more, and that would have had only one outcome, which would not have been a good one. So although I have made many mistakes in my life, I am proud to be able to say that getting into drugs was not one of them.

Apart from the drugs, when we were on board the yachts it was common to see guns and various other firearms lying all over the place, as well as huge wads of cash. I suppose that I could have pocketed thousands if I had wanted to, and it wouldn't have been missed, but they were lavishing thousands on me anyway, and I was earning such great money on my own that it never once entered my head.

The guns were something entirely different though. Again through my Dad, I knew the damage that guns could cause, and I knew that the type of men who carried them were not the sort that you would ever consider taking home to meet Mummy and Daddy, especially when Daddy was a high-ranking detective in the Met. With all the drugs and the drink, it would have been all too easy for things to get out of hand, for an argument, or even a mild disagreement, to end up with somebody pointing a gun, pulling the trigger and blowing somebody's brains out. All they would have had to do was go upstairs and throw the body overboard.

I look back upon it now and shudder, especially since I know how cheap life was to these men – or at least the lives of the girls such as myself that they treated like playthings. Do you think that any of them would have lost even one minute's sleep if anything had happened to any of us? Of course not.

So I knew that I had to play the game and keep my mouth shut. I don't suppose that I was truly aware of the danger I could have been in at that time – it wasn't until much later when I sat down and thought it through that I realised how vulnerable I had been.

You might be surprised to learn, by the way, that when I told my parents I'd landed a job as a Bunny Girl, they were actually very proud of me. Mum was pleased I'd got off my backside and found some work and although Dad would probably have preferred that I was working in an office, I think that because the Playboy Club had a swanky Park Lane address then he assured himself that it must be all legal and above board. And I am sure that he would have checked the place out with his colleagues, who would have told him it was frequented by rich Arabs and celebrities.

Or maybe Dad just turned a blind eye to it all. He would also have known that although I was something of a wild child, I would never do anything that I didn't want to do. He would also have convinced himself that I would never allow myself to be put in a dangerous position – such as being on a yacht with men who were armed and stoned out of their brains on cocaine. No, I would never do that! My mother had probably given up on me by that time, so any job would do.

Film stars and television celebrities would frequent the club, but I was never much impressed by celebrity. Yes, I knew who they were, but they were just normal human beings, made of flesh and bone. I was never one to jump up and down with excitement if somebody like Michael Caine or Omar Sharif walked in, although many of the girls I worked with would swoon at the very sight of a famous actor. As far as I was concerned, the only difference between us was that they had pots of money.

And I was never especially impressed by the footballers who appeared. They didn't have the money that today's players have, but some of them were great fun, and some of them were very good looking. There was one in particular that I had a brief encounter with when I went to work at another club, but more of that later.

During one lunchtime shift at the club I had been told to go for a break. I would normally have used the staff toilets but on this occasion I used the same ladies' toilets that the customers would use and when I walked in I stopped dead in my tracks. There in the corner were a man and a woman. She was on all fours with her knickers down around her ankles, and he was on all fours behind her snorting cocaine from her bare backside.

For a moment or two they were completely oblivious to me. I didn't know how I was supposed to react. A lot of women would have screamed and run out of the toilets, but I couldn't quite believe what I was seeing. Suddenly, the man realised there were somebody else in the toilet and he looked up at me.

What should I do? Well, I had come into the ladies for a reason, so I found a cubicle and in I went. When I emerged, the woman was standing in front of the mirror trying to put her lipstick on, but she was so stoned that she was incapable of doing it.

The man simply smiled, and said in an American accent: "Do you want to join us, baby?"

"Do I want to join you? Do I want to join you in what precisely?"

By this time, he had pulled the woman back towards him and, unbelievably, she got down on all fours again and pulled up her skirt and he bent down and starting kissing her between her legs and snorting off the rest of the coke. It was easily the most bizarre thing that I had ever witnessed, and I had seen some pretty strange things in my life. I also found it quite extraordinary that something that should have been happening in the privacy of a bedroom was actually being played out on the floor of the ladies' toilets – I was sure they had seen some things over the years, but this was surely a first, even for the Playboy.

Then he got up and started walking towards me. It was clear that he was now more interested in me than he was in his companion but I told him that I was on a break and that I had to go back to work. And that was when it dawned on me. The man standing in front of me, who had moments earlier been cavorting on the floor of the ladies' toilets in the Playboy Club in Park Lane was Telly Savalas, one of the most instantly recognisable actors on the planet. At the time he was starring in the incredibly popular TV detective series *Kojak*, in which his catchphrase was: "Who loves ya, baby?" A little bit different to: "Do you want to join us, baby?", I am sure you will agree.

He seemed only mildly put out that I had interrupted his fun, but I figured that was only because he was concerned that I might go and tell somebody. I am certain that if I had given him even the slightest encouragement, he would quite happily have had me sprawled all over the floor too, but there was no way I was going to allow that to happen. We hadn't even been properly introduced, for goodness sake!

I made my excuses and left, thinking that I would never see him again, but it turned out that he was filming in London and he became a frequent visitor to the club. He always sought me out, and eventually he asked me if I would go out with him for a coffee. Telly Savalas was not an attractive man, and he was well into his fifties when I knew him. But he had that special thing that some human beings possess – charisma. And when he asked me out there was never going to be any way that I could refuse him.

He was utterly charming, despite his part-time cocaine habit. We would go for coffee at the cafe in Park Lane. Before long, the inevitable happened and we became lovers. Savalas always stayed at the Inn At The Park Hotel when he was in London, and that was usually where we would end up. He loved women and he adored being the centre of attention, but the thing was that he preferred threesomes to one on one, and so it was that I ended up making love with him and another woman.

Whenever we were out, he would always open doors for me and he was really polite but, like the Arabs I talked about before, he was after something.

He was one of those men who got on off on excitement, but so did I, and the thrill of possibly being caught (as I had witnessed with my own eyes). He would follow me into the toilet when we were out and loved having a quick grope and a snog, and when I was in work he would also follow me into the loo and got off on sticking his fingers up my fanny. And then he would head off to the tables and gamble. Savalas was a big gambler, and he didn't mind losing money. Mind you, back in those days he was earning a fortune.

Remember, too, that he had starred in a lot of major movies, films that grossed vast sums at the box office – *Battle Of The Bulge*, *The Dirty Dozen*, *Escape From Athena*, *Kelly's Heroes*. He played macho characters, and that is the way he was in real life.

My relationship with him lasted for months, but the funny thing is that I never considered myself to be his girlfriend. It was all about sex, and sex for Telly Savalas was all about getting it on with two or three beautiful women, and then he would move on to the next ones. But he kept coming back for more.

Sometimes he would turn up at the Playboy Club and tell me he wanted me to go with him right there and then, so I would go and see the boss and pretend to be feeling ill – as long as the club wasn't too busy, they would tell me I could go, and off we would head to the Inn In The Park.

Going out for dinner? Heading off to a nightclub? Joining him for a quiet drink? No, not really. It was just about sex. Sometimes he got so desperate that he would grab hold of me and we would end up doing it outside the ladies' toilets. Anybody could have caught us, but he didn't care. I suppose his view was that he was a big Hollywood star and he could always buy off anybody who threatened to cause trouble for him.

Eventually, of course, he returned to the United States, although I would bump into him again some years later at another club where I worked, the Barracuda, when he walked in with his brother, George – you have never in your life seen two brothers who looked more different than those two. George had this thick mop of curly hair and was, well, fat, while Savalas shaved his head and looked after his physique.

Paul McCartney was another regular at the Playboy, as was John Lennon before he went to live in New York.

And then there was the Arab who threatened to throw acid in my face. How on earth did I allow myself to get into that position? This was a man I had a fling with, and who later told me that he wanted me to donate my eggs to his wife, who was sterile. I refused, and his solution was to threaten to disfigure me with acid. Charming, eh?

To start at the beginning, I met him at the club and he was loaded. Now there is wealthy and there is super-wealthy, and this guy fell into the latter category. And everywhere he went, his bodyguards went too.

Well, not quite everywhere, but you get the picture.

He went out of his way to woo me and I fell for him, hook, line and sinker. I thought that I was in love with him, and I thought that he loved me. And I had no idea whatsoever that he was married. I suppose the dream of most of the Bunny Girls was that they would meet a millionaire who whisk them away to a new life, and for some, that dream did come true. I am sure that some of the girls even loved the men they went off with. And who knows? One or two of the men may even have loved the girls in return. But not many. They were playthings, to be discarded and thrown out with the rubbish when they were no longer needed.

Let's call him Mohammad. Everything I wanted, this man gave me. We went to the best restaurants in London and he bought me the finest jewellery and the most expensive designer clothes. It didn't take long for me to fall for him, and it wasn't just about the money either. This was a man you would want to take home to meet your parents, right up until the moment he sat me down and said: "Sarah, I want you to donate your eggs for my wife so that she can have a baby. I will see to it that you are well rewarded."

Well rewarded? Who the hell did he think that he was talking to? His pet dog. I was devastated.

"You didn't tell me you were married, you bastard."

"It is of no concern to you Sarah. She is my wife, she is sterile and I want a son or a daughter."

And then I found myself feeling sorry for him and asking how I could help. The next thing was that I was at the Wellington Hospital, being interviewed by a surgeon who wanted an assurance that I was not being paid for donating my eggs.

"To receive payment is illegal, but it is perfectly all right for you to donate your eggs as a gift," he explained. "You should also understand that this is not a straightforward procedure [remember that we are talking about 1977] and you could be left with a small scar."

"A scar? Nobody said anything to me about a scar."

Alarm bells were ringing in my brain. Mohammad had told me that after I'd donated eggs, our relationship would continue as it had before. In the meantime I had to go back to the hospital several times and underwent several interviews and suchlike, and the longer it all went on, the more uneasy I began to feel. Why the hell was I giving my eggs to the wife of the man I was having an affair with? And I had never met this woman – what's more, he made it clear that he didn't want me to meet her.

I woke up one day and it was as if somebody had switched on a light. I made up my mind that I wasn't going to go through with it, and I told him so. To say that he was not a happy Arab is the understatement of all time. He was furious.

"I told you I would look after you, and I am a man of my word. It will be fine. You will be fine," he said.

But this was my body. Early in our relationship, I'd confided in Mohammad that I was only 17 when I started working for the Playboy Club and he threatened to spill the beans, saying that if they found out I be sacked on the spot. And then he delivered the coup de grace, saying he would throw acid in my face if I didn't do what he wanted. If ever I needed confirmation that he didn't give a toss about me, he had just proved it.

I decided to call his bluff and told him to do whatever he wanted. Big mistake. I turned up for work one day, was summoned to the Bunny Mother's office and given my marching orders, ostensibly because I had lied about my age, but in fact because he had told a pack of lies about me and it was easier for to get rid of me than to risk upsetting one of the biggest and best customers.

This was a man I'd looked upon as my knight in shining armour. And so ended another chapter in my life. I'd been at Playboy for 18 months and enjoyed almost every moment of it, and the ironic thing was that I was now old enough to work there legally. But I was out on my bunny ears.

CHAPTER SEVEN
Taken For A Ride

I had to find another job. It simply wasn't an option to sit around because I didn't have any money. Yes, I had lots of great clothes and some fabulous jewellery, but I had managed to fritter away almost all of the money I earned. Well I was young, and there was no way that I was ever going to open a savings account – that was something your parents did.

I decided to register with an employment agency that specialised in placing secretaries, even though I didn't possess a single relevant skill. I couldn't type and I didn't do shorthand, but I could answer a phone, and I could sit at a desk and look pretty. And the way I looked at it, what else did a secretary have to do?

The day I went to the agency I was told to sit down and somebody effectively gave me a formal interview. The first question they asked was: "What speed is your shorthand?" I stared back blankly before replying: "I don't do shorthand."

"Fine. What about your typing then? What speed do you type at?"

"I don't type either."

"Fine." It wasn't fine though. She was clearly wondering what the hell I was doing registering with a secretarial agency when I didn't possess the two most basic skills. "To be honest Sarah, there doesn't seem to be much point in us taking your details. As a matter of interest, what was your last position?"

"I was a Bunny Girl."

By now she was struggling to remain patient with me, and I could hardly blame her.

"A Bunny Girl? And why did you leave?"

"I was fired because I was under age when they first took me on."

Secretaries were meant to be paragons of virtue, the soul of discretion, and I guess that wasn't really me.

"So you can't type, you don't do shorthand and you were sacked from your last job. What can you do?"

"Well I can speak nicely and I can answer the phone."

"Mmm, well that's always something, I suppose."

She was also pretty impressed when I told her that I used to work at the Alexon Fashion House and that I had done a bit of switchboard work while I was there. Things were looking up, and she was actually starting to take a note of some of my details.

Her parting shot was: "I don't know if there is going to be anything much for you, but I will let you know if anything comes up."

I wasn't hopeful.

A few days later, out of the blue, I got a phone call from the agency to tell me that they might have something for me after all, that somebody was starting a business in Pimlico (near Victoria Station, if you can believe it) and that he was looking for a secretary, and wasn't too bothered whether or not she could type or do shorthand. Was I interested? Of course I was.

I will never forget the first time that I met Michael Rutt. The day I went to meet him for my job interview I was wearing a white skirt, a white top and no bra – the rain was coming down in stair-rods and, of course, I had no umbrella with me. By the time I got to his office, which was in a basement, I was drenched.

Rutt was short, fat balding man who chain-smoked French cigarettes and walked like James Cagney. I was ushered into what he called his den, which had no windows and a bolt on the door. Once he had shown me in, he closed the door and bolted it, and told me to sit on a sofa that seemed to fill the room.

I should have been worried about being locked in a room with a complete stranger, but I wasn't concerned. Naturally, I apologised to him for my appearance and he said: "Don't worry about it Sarah, you look just great to me."

He then asked if I wanted a drink. I assumed he meant a tea or a coffee, so I said yes. He poured out a whisky for himself and asked me what I fancied so I asked for a vodka and tonic. When he handed it to me, I took a sip and thought that my head was going to blow off. Talk about strong! This was like rocket fuel. How much vodka had he put in?

Let's just say that the interview that followed was not the most conventional. We ended up talking about my time at the Playboy Club and I told him about some of the adventures I'd had. He said nothing about any secretarial duties; in fact, he said nothing at all about the job I had come for. We just sat and talked and drank.

I had half an eye on the bolted door, and although I knew it wasn't normal to be locked in an office with a stranger, I was certain that I could get out whenever I wanted. In the end, I was with him for hours, getting steadily more and more pissed. Every so often he would get up, unbolt the door and go to the toilet, so if I had wanted to get out that would have been the time to do it, but I was having a good time.

I had to go to the toilet too, and each time I came back into the room he would get up and bolt the door closed again. And still there was no talk about a job.

Eventually he told me that he ran an overseas property development company and that he had taken on several salesmen that he had known for many years. "Basically, we sell property abroad," he said.

"It all sounds fine Michael, but are you going to talk to me about the job you would want me to do? Are you going to give me the job?"

"You want the job even though you don't know what it is? Tell you what, show us your tits and the job is yours."

In a split second I thought to myself: "What's a girl to do? I need a job, he is offering me a job, and all he wants in return is some kind of sexual gratification." Without any hesitation, I lifted my top.

"You've got fabulous tits Sarah."

"Tell me something I don't know. Why do you think they took me on as a Bunny Girl?"

As I was talking to him I walked over to him. He was sitting in a chair on wheels, and I reached forward, unzipped his trousers to reveal an erect penis and I thought to myself: "Ah well, in for a penny, in for a pound." With that, I straddled him and sat on his cock, still with my breasts exposed. We had sex and, with that, he told me that the job was mine. "Don't worry about the fucking job kid. Just come into the office every day, look good and answer the phone, say, 'Hello, Laird and Co', and take down any details for me. I will attend to it all when I get in."

And that, ladies and gentlemen, was my introduction to one Michael Rutt. The job was as advertised on the tin, or so I thought, and he used to wander into the office each day at about 11am, go into his den and go through his paperwork while drinking a coffee laced with Carnation milk. By lunchtime the coffee was laced with whisky, and by early afternoon he was calling me into the office, bolting the door and demanding sex with me. And I was happy to oblige.

He was in his forties and he was married with a young son, and I would end up babysitting for them. It was bizarre.

While I was working for Michael Rutt, I entered the Miss Bromley beauty contest. I am sure that I don't have to paint a picture for you – it was all pretty tawdry, with a host of girls having to parade in swimsuits in front of a lot of lecherous men, with the promise of a few quid for the winner, perhaps the chance of a modelling contract and the opportunity to go on to compete in Miss England, Miss United Kingdom and then, of course, Miss World. Yeah, right.

Right up until about an hour before the thing started, I wasn't sure if I wanted to go through with it, but eventually I thought: "You are doing nothing else tonight girl, so let's go along and see what happens."

I put a tight black dress and made up my hair in the style of Marilyn Monroe. Even though I say it myself, I looked pretty hot, but because I had procrastinated so much, I arrived at the last moment. I later discovered that the judges had been trying to get it on with all the other girls. Why? Because if they indicated that they might be prepared to sleep with a judge then it would improve their chances. Let's be clear what we are talking about here – if you agreed to bring a smile to the face of one of the judges, you would have a better chance of winning...Miss Bromley!

I would have revelled in the opportunity to wrap the judges around my little finger and flirt with them, but I couldn't because I hadn't given myself enough time. It meant that, although I didn't know it, I had absolutely no chance of winning.

There was a part where you were interviewed and had the opportunity to talk about yourself, and I was good at that. They struggled to get me to shut up, but I knew that if I could show something of my personality, as well as something of my body, then I might have proper chance of winning. If I try my hand at something, I don't do it to finish second.

I put on my best possible voice, and talked about my fascination for American sports car – I was making it all up as I was going along, of course. I had the compere eating out the palm of my hand and I thought that I had the contest in the bag. None of the other girls could string more than a couple of words together.

But I didn't win. I finished runner-up, and I was livid. The local newspaper took a photograph and it was pretty obvious to anybody who saw it that I was not a happy bunny. I looked at the girl who had won it and couldn't believe she had beaten me, so I stormed off and sat down in a sulk.

A few moments later I was approached by a man who said to me: "You should have won that." I agreed with him.

"But I know what you would be good at," he said. "You would make an amazing Page Three girl."

My ears pricked up because I knew that Page Three girls earned lots of money. He told me that he was a photographer, that he could help me if I was interested, and he handed me his business card and told me to phone him if I wanted him to take some pictures of me.

I swallowed it hook, line and sinker and phoned him a couple of days later and arranged to go to his studios in Farringdon. I had never met this man before, but I didn't take anybody with me.

I had brought some changes of clothes with me and he started snapping away, suggesting that I take this off and that off. Before I knew what was going on, I was topless, but it really didn't bother me. Besides, if I was going to become Britain's top Page Three girl then I was going to have to get used to posing semi-naked.

"Sarah, how about we do some shots with you taking your knickers off," he said. For the first time, alarm bells began to ring in my head. "What am I doing here with a photographer that I don't know, wearing next to no clothes?" I suddenly realised how vulnerable I was. And why, if he was taking photos of me for use as possible Page Three shots, would he want me to take everything off?

Next, he said that he wanted me to remove my knickers and lie back with my legs open. "I don't want to do that," I said. "You asked me here to do Page Three pictures. I am not interested in doing top shelf stuff. It doesn't interest me."

"Okay," he said, and off he went. Then I heard water running and a few moments later he asked me to come through and there in front of me was a bath full of hot soapy water. "Why don't you get in here then, Sarah. We've got all these bubbles, so there is no chance of anybody seeing anything you don't want them to see."

That didn't seem so bad, so I agreed, but I kept my knickers on. He carried on taking pictures and the next thing I knew was that he had removed all of his clothes and joined me in the bath. He started off trying to take a few more pictures, and then he produced a sponge and started to wash me, kiss me and touch me up. It was madness, but I had read all about the casting couch, so I just let him get on with it, thinking that maybe I had to do this to get to where I needed to be.

Afterwards, he promised that he would approach the likes of *The Sun* and *The Daily Mirror* with the photos he had taken, and he assured me that the offers of work would come pouring in. Guess what? I never heard from him again.

I wondered if there was even any film in the camera?

Amazingly, I wasn't put off for life by that experience, and some time later *The Mirror* ran a competition to find a new pin-up girl. Back then, they didn't feature pictures of topless girls, but they were what is called in the trade 'scantily-clad'.

"I can do that," I thought. There was an entry form to be filled in, accompanied by a photograph, and not long afterwards they contacted me and said that they wanted me to have my photograph taken.

This was all very different from the photographer in Farringdon. This time, there was a make-up girl who made sure that looked just so before sending me through to meet the photographer, Kent Gavin, who was one of the most famous of all Fleet Street photographers. He chatted away throughout the session and managed to make me feel at ease – he told me that I was a natural and that he really liked the way I looked.

It finished up with him telling me that *The Mirror* would be in touch if they wanted to take things further. If was the classic 'don't call us, we'll call you'. And they never did.

And so it was back to the day job with Michael Rutt. There was always lots of money, mostly in the form of cheques that had been paid to him as deposits for the overseas property that people thought they were buying. As far as I was concerned, it was all legal and above board and Michael Rutt was a successful businessman.

He advertised in the *Evening Standard* and in the national press, and the business poured in, with his salesmen being sent out to speak to potential customers.

The salesmen would come into the office from time to time and as I got to know them so I realised that each and every one of them had spent time in prison. It seemed that Michael was doing his bit for the rehabilitation of offenders. Very noble.

It would later emerge, of course, that the whole thing was just a massive con. There were no overseas properties – well there certainly weren't as many as Michael and his crew were selling.

One of the salesmen was a guy called Frank, and even Rutt was scared of this man. I later learnt that he had some serious connections in the underworld and was not an individual to be messed with. There was another salesman called Tony Brown with whom I ended up having an affair – I was 19 and he was about 42.

I took Tony home to meet my parents. He was older than my Mum and just a year or so younger than Dad. My father refused to talk to him and although my mother at least made an effort, she told me later that she thought it was disgusting that a man of that age would want to go out with a teenage girl. During that first meeting, I remember Mum asking Tony what the two of us were doing that weekend, and he replied: "We are going to stay in a hotel." That's right Tony, why don't you just spell it right out for my mother?

Tony lived in a flat not far from Notting Hill and one of his neighbours was a blonde lad called Gordon Sumner who lived with a woman called Frances Tomelty. One day I was in bed having sex with Tony, and he had invited Gordon to come down for a few drinks. A few more people arrived, one thing led to another, and before we knew where we were, there was a party going on. Gordon was in the process of putting a band together at the time – you may have heard of them. The called themselves The Police, and he became rather better known as Sting. Frances Tomelty was his first wife. Just so that there is no misunderstanding about this, Sting and I did not have sex, but we were in the same flat together when I was having sex with Tony.

Back at the office, they were generating so much 'business' that Michael had to hire a proper secretary, but he kept me on the payroll too. I say he hired a secretary, but he actually went though quite a few. He would devise errands for the secretary, designed to get her out of the office, or he would tell her to go and have a really long lunch, and while she was away I would be called into the den for sex. You could set a watch by it.

Sometimes I just wasn't in the mood for it and would tell him so, but he was never impressed. "What do you think I am paying your for?" he would shout. "Just get in here and get your knickers off." He had a foul temper and if I didn't please him he would throw the bottle of whisky at the wall. While it had been fun at the start, it all started to wear a bit thin after a while. I really didn't need that.

And while he might have thought he was the boss, I was actually quite a manipulative so-and-so. He used to pay me £200, cash in hand. Nobody I knew earned that sort of money. Remember that this was more than 30 years ago. When I needed or wanted to, I could wrap him round my little finger. I would ask him if he could lend me some money and it was always the same discussion: "Have you spent all your wages already kid?"

"Yes Michael," I would lie, and he would hand over a pile of cash, sometimes as much as £300. He would always say that he would dock it from my wages, but he was always pissed when I asked him for cash, so he forgot. As far as I was concerned, I was doing a job of work, and I was determined that I was going to be as well rewarded for it as possible.

He could be violent and aggressive. Usually it was brought on by drink, but sometimes he lost the plot when he was unable to perform sexually – and, of course, the reason that he sometimes couldn't was because he had drunk too much. I didn't help matters, I don't suppose, by shouting off my mouth when he wasn't able to perform. He pinned me up against the wall and threatened me on more than one occasion. It also frightened him that my Dad was a chief inspector in the police force. When we first got together he didn't know that, but it was only natural that it would come out in conversation at some point.

At one stage he tried to befriend my father, offering to take him to boxing matches and suchlike. I guess he must have thought that Dad would be a useful ally to have on his side should he ever need to call on him. But Dad was too cute to get caught out like that.

I also remember having a discussion with my mother during which I revealed that Michael sometimes scared me. Her response? "Well Sarah, you've got to have a job. Just try to make sure that you don't upset him, that's all."

Was this really what I wanted to be doing with my life? And although I might not be the brightest light in the house, I was also starting to feel a trifle uneasy about the business, about what Michael and his associates were actually doing. The money he was using to pay my wages, and the cash he handed over when I asked him for a sub, it was his punters' money.

He would take people on inspection flights to Spain and when they got there they would be met by somebody that Michael had on the payroll and off they would go to look at plots of land, upon which Michael would tell these innocent people that he had permission to build villas, flats, apartments. In reality, he didn't own the land and he had no permission to build anything. The entire thing was a con, designed to relieve people of as much money as possible, as quickly as possible. I guess that the plan was always for Michael and his associates to disappear in a puff of smoke before they were rumbled. It was despicable.

It was a house of cards, and it was inevitable that it would come crashing down at some point.

There was one poor man, a Mr Wright, who paid a huge deposit based on the plot and plans he had been shown during his first inspection flight. The problem for Michael was that Mr Wright decided to fly back out to Spain to check on progress and, of course, there was no progress. Michael told him that he needed to pay more money. Unbelievably, he agreed to hand it over.

I wasn't party to these negotiations, so I don't know how much money was changing hands.

Alarm bells rang when I would open a letter and it would refer to the sale of a plot of land that I knew had already been sold to somebody else. I tried to put it down to an administrative error and convinced myself that really everything would be fine. Whenever I would draw Michael's attention to this he would simply say: "Don't worry about it kid. Don't worry about it. It's all fine." So I wouldn't worry about it.

Did I mention that Michael used to bring prostitutes back to the office at night? The way I looked at it was that it saved me a job, but his office was always disgusting after they had gone. There would be dirty glasses, empty spirit bottles and used condoms left on the floor. And yours truly had to clean it all up first thing most mornings.

I got friendly with one of the prostitutes, a girl called Penny and I ended up confronting Michael. "You are sleeping with her, aren't you?"

"Of course I'm not sleeping with her. She's a bloody prostitute and she's into drugs and God knows what else – I haven't a clue what she might have, and there's no way I am going to risk catching anything from her."

"Well how do you explain all the used condoms then?"

"Oh that's nothing to do with Penny. That's Borjana." Borjana was a Polish prostitute. So he was happy enough to admit that he was doing the deed with one whore, just not this other one. If I am truthful, I was jealous because, in my own way, I loved Michael Rutt. I can't half pick them.

His life was all about screwing prostitutes, knocking off his secretary and extracting money from innocent people, and I had become a part of it. And all because I refused to donate eggs to an Arab's wife!

Inevitably, people came to the office, either to complain about lack of progress with their properties or to find out how the 'builders' were getting on. That's when I realised why he had a bolt on the door. I lost count of the number of times they would arrive when the two of us were in the den having it away. "Hello, Mr Rutt, are you there?" And we would have to hurriedly get dressed and make ourselves look respectable before opening the door to the client.

He had this amazing gift for being able to switch on and off, and suddenly he would be all business-like and would say to me: "Right then Sarah, go and get the paperwork for Mr Wright please. Mr Wright, please do take a seat and we will be with you right away."

I would dig out the file, return to the office and on more than one occasion I would be agog as he would say: "Mr Wright, I am going to leave you in Sarah's more than capable hands as I have a business meeting to go to. Sarah will tell you everything that you need to know. Good day." And with that he would be gone. The first time he did it I didn't have a clue what to do or say, but eventually I developed a way of telling them what I thought they wanted to hear.

The problem was that I ended up giving these people the impression that I was an integral part of the business, and if that were true then it would also make me part of the con. The truth is that I was as much an innocent victim in that part of things as they were. Yes I had my suspicions, but I was 19 years old and I was being paid good money. It was in my interests to turn a blind eye, to keep my head down and hope that it would all be okay.

I became a master of fobbing people off. I would tell them that there was a problem with our man in Spain, that he'd had a death in the family and had been away from the site. Or I would tell them that there had been a delay with supplies because of a strike. Anything to appease them. Then I would take a note of their number and promise to get back to them just as soon as I heard back from Spain.

Eventually, Michael started taking me on flights to Spain with him, and I would carry a bag full of money for him on each trip. I don't know what he did with it when we got there, although I guess that he must have had Spanish bank accounts, and I don't know how much money he was asking me to carry, but I do know that it wasn't petty cash.

We used to do this once every six weeks or so. I used to worry about walking through customs carrying a holdall full of cash but I was never once challenged. Security back in those days was pretty lax, to say the least.

He told me not to ask any questions, so I didn't. Everything happened in Sitges in Spain. We would arrive at the hotel where we stayed and he would tell me to get in a car at a specific time, go to a specific meeting place – usually a dusty layby in the middle of nowhere - and hand over the bag to somebody that I can only describe as a former boxer with his nose wrapped halfway round his face. Not somebody that you would want to engage in polite conversation or take home to meet Mummy. By now I knew that I was involved in something that I shouldn't be. This was not normal behaviour.

I would hand the bag over and get a parcel in return. I never looked inside because I didn't want to consider what I might be carrying. I would then get back into the car, drive straight back to the hotel, give Michael the parcel and head down to the pool and sunbathe. A few minutes later he would join me, hold hands and make like we were holidaymakers. I managed to persuade myself that we were having a break, just like normal tourists.

But normal tourists didn't hold meetings in hotel rooms, and normal tourists didn't tell their girlfriends to make themselves scarce while those meetings were going on.

I was with Michael Rutt for four years – that is a hell of a time to keep all those plates spinning and remain one step ahead of the authorities. But somehow he managed to do it. He drove around in a Rolls-Royce, so that should give you some idea of the sort of money he was making.

As time past, so the pressure began to increase. Whereas the meetings he used to hold with his salesmen in the early deals had been pretty relaxed affairs, now he was shouting and swearing at them, telling them they had to secure this deal or that deal. I guess that the vultures were closing in and that Michael could see the writing on the wall. I even heard him threatening to shoot one of them.

It had to come to end, and it did. In the most spectacular fashion. One of Michael's customers realised he was being taken for a ride and tried to get his money back. When he couldn't get any satisfaction he got in touch with ITN and the next thing we knew was that Roger Cook, the world renowned investigative journalist, came crashing into the office.

Lots of people had been complaining. Michael had stopped coming into the office, and he was no longer paying me, but I kept turning up for work because I felt that I owed him that. It all meant that I was usually the only person in the office.

We had no idea, but Cook and his team had been watching us for days, perhaps even for weeks. When the whole thing broke on the news it quickly became obvious that they had had us all under observation. It was actually pretty scary.

One day Cook knocked on the door. There was just him and a cameraman. I recognised him immediately. A camera was thrust in my face and Cook said: "I am Roger Cook from ITN. Is Michael Rutt in?"

"No, he isn't here."

"Well we want to interview him about his overseas property development that doesn't exist and the poor unsuspecting victims who have been conned out of hundreds of thousands of pounds. Do you know anything about it?"

"I am just a secretary," I managed to blurt out. "I don't know what you are talking about."

With that, I closed the door and away he went. I then phoned Michael to warn him. But Cook managed to track him down and on the news later that night there he was, again with the camera in Michael's face, and Michael was giving him a mouthful of abuse, telling him he had nothing to say.

Michael was charged with fraud and ended up going to trial at the Old Bailey. But before that, I felt that the guy needed my help so I still kept going into the office to answer the phones and field the crap. Obviously he wasn't paying me but I figured that I had earned a lot of money with him and he needed my help.

He was given bail and he used to come into the office from time to time but finally the time came for his trial. It seemed to go on for ever and then I was called to appear, effectively as the star witness for the prosecution. I was the only one who could tell the whole story.

My Dad was worried about how I was going to be treated. He was based at Scotland Yard at the time, but he had worked for the Fraud Squad and had a lot of contacts, people he spoke to in the run-up to the trial. He wanted to ensure that I wasn't going to be stitched up, that they would be fair with me.

He told me that I had nothing to worry about. I wasn't so sure.

I realised that I had two ways of dealing with things. I could either go in and act the air-headed blonde bimbo or I could give them everything they wanted to hear. The thing is that I felt loyalty towards Michael and, to be frank, I was worried that if he felt I was responsible for having him sent down then he might have me beaten up, or worse. So I opted for the air-head approach.

I played it thick, as thick as two short planks. I ended up having them in hysterics, right from the off. I was asked to take the oath and put my hand on the Bible, but told them that I didn't know if I could do it because I didn't believe in God. "That is immaterial Miss Goddard, you have to swear on oath. You have no choice."

The prosecutor was very aggressive towards me, but I had been warned to expect that. He asked me how I would describe Mr Wright, the aggrieved customer to whom I referred earlier. "He was aggressive and mean," I replied.

"No Miss Goddard, I don't mean that. I mean, how would you describe his relationship with Michael Rutt?"

And then he tried to tackle me about the finances. "Did you know that Michael Rutt was committing fraud?"

"Of course not. I was his secretary."

"Cheques came into the office every day and you banked them Miss Goddard. Where did you bank them?"

"I didn't bank them. I had nothing to do with the cheques."

That part was true. Michael used to take the cheques away, bank them, wait for them to clear and then appear with huge wads of cash.

"What do you know about Mr Rutt's banking procedures"

"I don't know anything about that. I just know about all the wanking that went on, and all the sex that happened in Michael's office."

There was a stunned silence in the court.

And so it went on. I knew that if I told them that Michael made me carry bags full of money to Spain for him then I would be the one who would be responsible for him being sent down, and I just couldn't bring myself to do that. If he was going down, it wasn't going to be because of any evidence that I gave.

In the end, they more or less gave up on me. It didn't do any good though. Michael was sent down for ten years, and as far as I am aware, none of the investors ever saw a penny of their money again.

While he was in prison, Michael's wife divorced him. I could have given up on him, too, but I didn't and I visited him several times.

I was probably the first person he contacted when he got out of jail, and it was to tell me that he had started an escort agency in Paddington Green. He called it Paramount and it turned out to be yet another knocking shop. It seemed that he had actually learnt very little while he had been locked up. He was sending girls out to have sex with complete strangers.

He asked me to come and see him and when I walked into his office there was a girl sitting there – as soon as he saw me he told her to clear off. It was like nothing had changed. "God, I've missed you kid," he said. "I've really missed you. Show us your tits!"

But by now I had grown up. Although he was sent down for ten years, Michael only served about seven. I looked at all the girls who were passing through his hands; they were very young and reminded me of how I had been on that wet day when I first walked into his office in the basement. I just felt that he was taking advantage of them and that was when I decided that there wasn't a future for us second time around.

I don't know if he wanted me to work with him because the discussion never took place. It was great to see him and I was delighted that he had got through the prison sentence in one piece. We kissed and he gave me the most enormous cuddle. I sat down and Michael went off to make us a cup of coffee. While he was gone, a young girl walked in and I asked her how old she was. She was just 17, and here she was effectively working as a prostitute.

"What are you doing here?" I asked her.

"I've come for a job," she replied.

"What sort of job is it going to be?"

"I think it involves doing some modelling and stuff like that, and going out with some men."

"Well you know what that means, don't you? You don't really want to be here, do you?"

I didn't realise that Michael was listening to every word, and he shouted: "Don't you dare start meddling in my affairs, Sarah. If she wants to come and work for me, she will come and work for me. Simple as that. It is lovely to see you again, but you can fuck off if you are going to start interfering with my girls."

I thought to myself: "You bastard. You haven't changed one bit. Seven years inside has taught you nothing. You are going to ruin these girls."

I wanted nothing to do with it. Don't get me wrong – if, years earlier, somebody had come along and tried to advise me against the path I was taking when I was with Jock, I wouldn't have paid any attention at all, so I knew that I was wasting my breath with Michael's girl. The difference was that this time I didn't have to hang around and watch it; I didn't have to be a part of it.

Michael asked me to help establish Paramount and I did work with him for a while, answering phones and getting punters in. He also used to send me out to meet what he regarded as his high-end customers. My job was to perform in a meet-and-greet capacity, and I never had sex with any of them.

Apart from anything else, I was married at the time and I had another job. As far as I was concerned, I was just helping him out for a while. He was also a good man to have on my side because I always knew that if I got into any trouble I could call on Michael and he would have it sorted it out for me.

Eventually it reached the point where my husband told me that if I continued to see Michael and work with him then our marriage would be over, and that is when I called it a day.

CHAPTER EIGHT
Here We Go Again

After Michael was locked up, I found myself without a job again. What could I do? I still wasn't trained to do much of anything, but I figured that I could call on the experience I had picked up at the Playboy Club.

I knew that I was good with people, and that men liked me, found me attractive and related to me, so maybe I could find bar work or land a job in a casino. I ended up working as a topless waitress in a nightclub called Toppers, in central London. I had never been too worried about showing off my assets, and it was explained to me that there was a strict 'hands off' policy, and that any customers who laid a finger on me or any of the other waitresses would be thrown out. I was proud of my body and was happy to show it off.

One of the first things that struck me about the place was that there was a really odd smell. I later discovered that it came from a red carpet onto which all the waitresses were encouraged to throw their champagne. A customer would buy you a glass of champagne and when he wasn't looking, we would tip it out on the carpet, so he would then feel obliged to buy another. It was a scam, designed to get the customers spending as much money as possible. But it was also designed to protect us because if we were pouring our champagne away then it meant we couldn't get drunk.

Every so often the cleaners had to spray the carpet with some sort of concoction to get rid of the smell of stale alcohol.

I had been interviewed by a woman called Denise, a beautiful raven-haired creature who was in charge of all the girls. During the interview she said: "You do realise that this is a topless club?" I told her that I did, and that I wasn't worried about that at all, and then she uttered the words I had heard so many times before: "Okay then Sarah, so I am going to have to ask you to show me your tits." They obviously passed the test because I got the job.

I started the next day and quickly realised that the rest of the girls I was working with were fairly rough and ready. As a result, they took an instant dislike to me. It didn't bother me, but it always makes life easier if you are popular. I suppose I stood out like a sore thumb once again because I spoke properly.

This place was nothing like the Playboy Club, where all the girls were beautiful. At Toppers, there were all shapes and sizes, and some of the women were not at all attractive. It would have been an act of kindness to have had them put down.

The way it worked was that all the girls would queue up, just like a cattle market, and customers would come in and choose the ones they wanted to spend time with. We would then go through to the bar and talk and drink with them (or pretend to drink with them, I should say).

I used to get tired of being asked the same old questions by these guys. It was a case of: "What's a nice girl like you doing in a place like this?" Sometimes I told them the truth and explained what had happened with Michael Rutt, and they would look at me in disbelief. So I would find myself spinning all sorts of stories to keep them entertained. Many of them would also insist on covering me up with their coats or jackets; I found this upsetting because, as I have already said, I had no issues with showing off my breasts. I am sure they felt that I needed to be protected, but I didn't. I chose to do the job, although it wasn't the most challenging work I have ever done. So I would find myself sitting talking to a man, with his jacket draped over my shoulders, and Denise would march over and tell me to take the jacket off.

"But I want her to put my jacket on."

"I am sorry sir, but we have rules, and one of the rules is that the girls must be topless at all times."

And off would come the jacket. Upstairs there was a room where some of the girls earned extra money by doing some private dancing, and I soon cottoned on to that. Dancing is one of my great passions, so this was a fun way to earn a few quid.

Before long, I found that I was in demand – and I tell you for nothing that my champagne didn't end up on the floor. What a shocking way to treat perfectly good alcohol.

Then I acquired a stalker. This same guy started coming in every night, and he would always ask for me and want me to do personal dances for him. I found him very creepy and I was uncomfortable with him. He also used to shower me with gifts, and he even bought me a car. It all came to a head when he asked me to marry him and I turned him down flat. One night I came out of the club and he was waiting for me. He pinned me up against the wall and threatened to kill me. He knew where I lived, so I decided it was time to move out of my flat, leave Toppers and find a new job.

Remember I mentioned an encounter with a famous footballer?

At about this time, George Best owned a nightclub called Blondes in Dover Street, London. My best friend, Karen Deacon, and I used to spend a lot of time drinking in Dover Street Wine Bar, and so did Best – in fact, he spent more time in the wine bar than he did in his own club, which was directly opposite.

It used to break my heart to see what had become of this gorgeous man. At one stage in his life he had it all, but by the 1980s he seemed to spend most of his life roaring drink. Every time we saw him he was propping up the bar, often barely able to string more than a couple of words together. And there were always hangers-on with him, as well as a never-ending queue of women.

I have never been star-struck, but there was something about George Best and one night I ended up talking to him after Karen decided to leave early and get a taxi home. I didn't home in on him or anything like – it just so happened that we were sitting next to one another at the bar.

I was talking and he was talking as well, but I couldn't understand a word – it was a combination of his Northern Irish accent, the fact that he'd had lots to drink and the background music.

He was such a flirt. Even while he was trying to chat me up, his eyes were darting around the bar at every other attractive woman. The evening ended with the two of us having sex in a back alley behind the wine bar. Talk about knowing how to show a girl a good time! It was quick and it was pretty much instantly forgettable – and, thankfully, it was never repeated.

I landed a position as a receptionist at the Sportsman Club in London's Tottenham Court Road. It was only part-time, but it was a start.

While I was there I met John Glen, who would become my first husband. He always used to play a trick on new receptionists, along the following lines. "Sarah, will you put out a call for a Mr Mike Hunt please to come to reception?"

I thought nothing of it, and duly switched on the microphone and bellowed: "Will Mike Hunt come to the front desk please?" Everybody fell about laughing and eventually the penny dropped with me too. Mike Hunt, my arse!

I took an instant dislike to John. He reminded me of the Honey

Monster, as wide as he was tall – and he was only a storeman. Before long he asked me out. I had to admit that he had some balls. He wasn't my cup of tea at all and I just thought he was a cheeky bastard with ideas above his station, but I eventually agreed to go out with him, more out of pity than anything else.

Apart from anything else, he didn't have two pennies to rub together.

I had made it clear to him that we were only going out for one drink. But one became two, two became three, three became four...and before I knew where I was, I was pissed again. John drank Jack Daniels and coke and he, too, could pack it away.

As the evening wore on, I found myself warming to him, and it had nothing to do with the booze. The fact of the matter was that John was one of the funniest men I had ever met, and he had me rolling about with laughter. So suddenly you don't notice the fact that the man sitting opposite is not exactly God's gift to women.

He would later say to me: "Basically Sarah, I have always felt that if I can make you laugh, then I can screw you." And he was right.

I enjoyed his company and for the first time in my life I was with a man who wasn't using me and it didn't take long for me to fall in love with him. In saying that, I have always been able to fall in love with people seemingly at the drop of a hat.

My position was that I needed a job and I needed somewhere to live, and I ended up living with him. To be more accurate, I ended up moving in with John and his parents in their council house in Bow, East London.

The Playboy Club, the fabulously rich Arabs, the clothes, the jewellery – it all seemed a million miles away from the life I was now leading. My parents had already made it clear to me that moving back in with them was not an option, so I had to try and make the best of what was clearly a pretty bad job. But I was happy.

I loved John's parents dearly. They would do anything for me, real salt of the earth people. I had only been used to dealing with people who wanted to use me, who wanted to take whatever they could get from me, but John's father would have given me his last penny. And the best thing of all was that he expected nothing in return.

All the while, I had this nagging feeling that this was not the lifestyle I wanted. Living in a council house was not for me.

I landed a job as a waitress at the Golden Nugget casino in Shaftesbury Avenue – it was owned by the same company that owned The Sportsman Club. The vast majority of customers were Chinese, and boy did they love gambling. They would bet on absolutely anything at all. And it was also used by lots of Americans.

From the day the Golden Nugget opened it was packed to the brim and we were rushed off our feet. John also managed to get a transfer to reception at the Golden Nugget, so the two of us were still working together and we were earning more money – not a fortune, obviously, but enough.

For me, all the Playboy memories came flooding back, and I used to make a point of carrying my tray in the most theatrical manner possible. I also used to flirt with all the customers, on the basis that they might give me a better tip if they thought there was any chance of getting off with me. And it worked.

I had to be totally focused on what I was doing, be pleasant to the punters, earn as much money as I could and then go home, satisfied that I had done the job to the best of my ability. The other girls hated me because I was good at what I did, which meant I always received better tips than anybody else. There was never any question of us having to share out our tips either – what you earned was yours. End of story.

And why would I want to give any of my hard-earned cash to girls who couldn't do their jobs properly? No way. The most lucrative area was always the blackjack table but the head waitress refused to put me on there, so I just used to clean up with the roulette customers instead. You had to know how to play the game, and I was one of the best.

I managed to pick up a bit of Mandarin and Cantonese and would go out of my way to try and converse with the customers. I wasn't fluent by any means, but they loved the fact that somebody had made an effort. It made them feel special, that we weren't just interested in relieving them of the contents of their wallets, although that was precisely what management and staff alike wanted to do.

The first night I ever worked there I earned £180, and nine months later that had risen to around £1,000 per night, tax free. Mind you, I had to do well on tips because the wages were awful. I can't remember the exact figure but it would have been something in the order of £30 per week.

I also have to say that it was fantastic to do a job, get well paid for it and not be expected to have sex with the customers.

We also used to have to do stints where we had to serve senior members of staff – the directors of the club. These guys were notorious for not tipping the girls, but I even managed to wrap them around my little finger too. I am not saying that I got anything like the same amount in tips when I served them, but I still managed to do well enough for myself, thank you very much.

How well did I do? Our first house in Leytonstone cost £27,000 and I paid for it myself, and didn't need a mortgage. That was a very special feeling. It took me less than six months to save the money.

John and I also got married. I had always dreamed of having a fabulous fairytale wedding, but the reality was rather different. We were married at a grotty registry office in Leytonstone. My Mum had met him and told me that I was making a huge mistake and that he was not the man who was going to make me happy. She was so convinced that she even threatened not to come to the wedding.

I managed to persuade her to change her mind, and in the end there were the two of us and our respective parents. We all went out for a meal, and that was it. That was my wedding day. Not at all what I'd had in mind for myself.

One evening I told him that I was going out for some fish and chips and when I came back I announced that I had been to a travel agent, and I had booked and paid for a two-week honeymoon in Crete. "When are we going?"

"Tomorrow."

I was beginning to feel restless so I started doing an embalming course. Don't ask! I have always been obsessed with death – it may have been something to do with my grandparents, because it seemed to be the only subject that they ever wanted to talk about. Mind you, that is quite common with older people, and I can only begin to imagine that it must have something to do with the fact that they become increasingly aware of their own mortality. As I sat and listened to these conversations I became fascinated by the entire subject of death. We would have family gatherings and would be sitting around the dining table and I cannot begin to tell you how many times the subject would come up. So it was always there, bubbling away in the back of my mind.

Dead bodies have never bothered me, but I have always been appalled at just how bad some corpses look. If you are going to see a loved one for the last time, you want to see them as they were before they died, not as if they have just been subjected to some bad cosmetic surgery. Or then there were the bodies that looked like ventriloquist's dummies. I mean, why would anybody slap a load of blusher on the face of a dead 80-year-old woman? But that is what was happening. There should be some dignity in death, both for the victims and for their families.

I offered my services to a number of funeral parlours, telling them that I would like to help apply make-up to the corpses, and they were happy to take me on. It was something I enjoyed doing because even going back to my days at theatre school, I had always had a talent for applying make-up. While I was applying the make-up, I would talk to the dead bodies, explaining to them what I was doing to them.

As I grew older, so I became interested in the entire embalming process and what was involved in making a dead body look presentable and acceptable to mourners. I began reading a host of books to learn about the entire procedure. The idea was that when I had got as much from the books as I could then I would embark on a proper practical course and learn everything there was to know about embalming.

It was an intense period in my life. I was working at the casino at night and during the day I was doing my thing at the funeral parlours and also fitting in my studies, and I was really enjoying it. When I set myself a target, I am like a machine, and I don't rest until I have achieved my goal.

But then I discovered that I was pregnant with Charlotte, my first daughter, and that put paid to that. I carried on working for a little while but I knew that I couldn't wander around in a skimpy costume at the casino when I was six or seven months pregnant. Apart from anything else, I astonished even myself by coming over all maternal; it wasn't something that I had expected, and I put it all down to my hormones. It felt good, and it felt entirely natural and comfortable to be pregnant, even though it wasn't planned.

I tried to convince myself that this was going to be the best baby in the world and that I was going to live happily ever after. And then I looked at John and found myself wondering what on earth I had let myself in for. Was I prepared to settle for this relationship?

John was a deeply intelligent man, but he had no ambition whatsoever. All these years later, he still lives in a council house. I believe that as you get older, you should become more ambitious.

When Charlotte was born, obviously I had to stay and home and look after her. There was no question of being able to go back to work at the casino, which meant that the only money that was coming in was what John was earning. Yes the house was paid for, but we still had all the bills to pay.

John liked a drink, so much so that when Charlotte was born he never came in to see me because he was out getting drunk with his mates, supposedly wetting the baby's head. To him, it might not have seemed terribly important, but I was hurt that he hadn't made the effort.

As the days turned into weeks our relationship became quite strained, not helped one bit by the fact that we were now struggling for money. He started drinking heavily and I was not fulfilled in any way. My life had turned from a glamorous existence where I could earn £1,000 a night to one where I was entirely dependent upon my husband for whatever handouts he put my way.

And I guess that he began to resent me because I started to put our daughter first, and he felt that I wasn't interested in him.

I was 24 years old and I kept thinking: "There has got to be more to life than this. This can't be what's in store for me for the rest of my life."

When I was pregnant I had felt so comfortable with it all that I started eating for England, with the result that I had put on five stones in weight. I was enormous and, as you can imagine, it was not something I enjoyed. I could not bear to look at myself in the mirror.

After Charlotte was born I worked hard to shed the excess weight, and then I worked even harder to get my shape back. Now I was ready to go back to work, and I managed to secure a job at our local wine bar in Leytonstone, which is where I met Glenn, the man who would turn out to be my second husband.

CHAPTER NINE
From The Frying Pan ...

Glenn Harvey was, and still is, an artist and was a regular customer in the wine bar. There was an instant attraction between the two of us and I guess it was inevitable that we would end up having an affair.

I am not ashamed of what Glenn and I did. My mother had been right about John – he was not the right man for me. Never was, never could be. Not in a million years. It was my fault as much as it was his, and when he asked me to marry him, I should have refused.

What can I tell you about Glenn? He was an incredibly gifted man, and he appeared to possess all the ambition that John lacked, but it turned out that he was all talk. He had lots of ideas, but never did anything about them, and was little more than a dreamer.

When he first swept me off my feet I convinced myself that he was a good catch. This was a man who worked as a graphic designer but who was a brilliant painter and caricaturist, a man who seemed to have the world at his fingertips. And he even had his own house.

We were great together sexually. He made me feel alive. I didn't realise it at the time, but I was probably suffering from post-natal depression. I certainly wasn't thinking straight, that's for sure.

The two of us had a whirlwind romance and I made up my mind that if Glenn asked me to live with him I would do so in a heartbeat. And when I did move in with him, I made the biggest mistake of my life – and I have made a few. I left Charlotte behind. I abandoned her.

Unsurprisingly, my parents disowned me, telling me that what I had done was disgusting and despicable. They wanted nothing to do with me. I could understand how they felt, but at no stage did they offer me help. I was desperately unhappy in my relationship with John and I needed a way out. Glenn offered me that escape route. But if my Mum and Dad had told me to come home, I would have done so in a flash and the relationship with Glenn might never have happened.

I know that I should have taken Charlotte with me, but I didn't, and it is something that I have had to live with ever since. Somehow, I managed to convince myself that she would be better off with John. There were also worries in the back of my mind about how Glenn would react to having a child in the house that wasn't his. You read some dreadful stories about the way that some stepchildren are treated.

But there was no way of sugar-coating it. Deep down, I knew that what I had done was terrible, and that the person who was most likely to suffer was going to be my daughter, who was an entirely innocent party in all of this. I used the fact that I'd let John carry on living in the house as a means of easing my conscience. In the end, I told him that if he gave me £5,000 he could keep the house, and that's what happened – it was a pretty poor investment on my return. Remember that I had paid £27,000 cash for the place, and it had rocketed in value.

In the end, I saw some sort of common sense, contacted John and we finally settled on an arrangement where I would have Charlotte at weekends.

He met another woman, Terry, and she eventually became pregnant but then had a miscarriage. As far as I was concerned, she was absolutely fine, but it turned out that nothing could have been further from the truth. I went round to the house one weekend to pick up Charlotte, as arranged, and there was no answer when I rang the doorbell. I was puzzled because I always picked her up at the same time, and they knew that. There were no mobile phones back then, so all that I could do was wait.

It seemed that I sat on the doorstep for hours, and as the time was passing I was beginning to feel uneasy. It turned out that John and Terry had disappeared and had taken Charlotte with them. The girlfriend had been desperate for a child of her own, and suffering the miscarriage had pushed her over the edge.

So now my daughter was missing. I was frantic. The worst thing of all was that I kept thinking that if I had not left her with John in the first place, none of this would have happened. It was my fault. Glenn told me it wasn't, but it was.

Days passed and we heard nothing. Then the days turned into weeks. By now I was at the end of my tether. Every time I switched on the news or picked up a newspaper I expected to hear or read about a young child being found dead.

Then, after three months, they were discovered in Bristol. John said that he had decided Charlotte would be better off being as far away from me as possible. He had heard that I was shagging around and made up his mind that I was a bad mother and that I had no right to have Charlotte under my roof. It had never occurred to him to pick up a telephone and tell me that my daughter was all right.

The police brought Charlotte back to me and then I decided to challenge him in court for full custody. He didn't turn up for the first court date, so they set a new one, and when he failed to appear for that one either, I was awarded full custody. And then I had to set about restoring my relationship with my daughter, hoping that no damage had been caused.

When the divorce from John came through, I was working at the

Barracuda Club. Glenn proposed to me and I dived straight into another marriage that was doomed to end in disaster. Glenn was a kind and loving man and he was brilliant with Charlotte, treating her as if she was his own child. It only made me realise once again what a huge mistake I had made in leaving her with John.

There was one big problem with our relationship, however – I have always loved excitement, even danger. I like to live on the edge, and for all that Glenn had these incredible artistic abilities, after a while I found him boring. Really, really boring. There was no spark.

There was also no money. Things were so bad that I had two pairs or shoes to my name – a black pair and a white pair. And I had hardly any clothes either.

On our first wedding anniversary I phoned him up to wish him a happy anniversary while I was in bed with an Arab I had met at the Barracuda.

CHAPTER TEN
Battered Beauty

When I started work at the Barracuda Club I was only doing two days a week. It was a casino, based in London, and it was another place that attracted that a great many high-rollers, people with more money than sense.

It was familiar territory for me, and it felt safe. I worked from 8pm until 4am. My job was to work on the switchboard, so I was basically just answering the phones. I was quite surprised to discover that all the other people who worked on the reception area were men – this was pretty unusual. Casinos would normally want to have a pretty face to greet customers as they arrived for the night. But not the Barracuda.

Over the course of my first couple of weeks I was introduced to all the reception staff and gradually got to know them all, but there was one who had been on holiday.

I am going to call him Faisal Mohamed - this is not his real name, but as you read on you will realise why I have given him an alias. He was born in Saudi Arabia and the first night the two of us were on duty together he walked up the stairs leading to the reception area, looked at me and said to the other guys: "Oh my God, and I've just got back together with my ex-wife." I thought he was an arrogant bastard, with his head stuck up his backside.

During the next couple of weeks he started sniffing around me. I knew that he fancied me, and I was flattered, even though I was married to Glenn and I also had Charlotte at home. If I'd had any sense at all, I would have kept him at arm's length, but that wasn't my style.

There is no point in denying it – I was attracted to the man. He had a magnetism, a great personality, although I would never have described him as being handsome. He possessed charisma. Unusually, he had red hair. By traditional Saudi standards, he was not a wealthy man, but he earned decent enough money.

One night after we finished work I couldn't get a taxi so he said he would give me a lift home, and I accepted. "Before I take you home, do you want to go on to a club?" he asked. I should have said no, but I didn't, so at four in the morning we ended up heading to a club for a drink. It turned out that he was also a fabulous dancer. This was the first time I had ever been with somebody who possessed a sense of rhythm – all my previous boyfriends and husbands hadn't the first idea; stick them on the dance floor and it was like dancing with your father at a family wedding.

But Faisal was different. He could really move, and that simply added to the attraction I felt for him. Nothing else happened that night. We had a drink and a few dances and then he took me home. He was the perfect gentleman.

Before I knew where I was, however, the two of us were having a full-blown affair. He lived in Portobello and I used to go back to his place when his wife was at work. It was all very messy, but I seemed to specialise in messy relationships at that point in my life. We had great sex, but our relationship wasn't just about what happened between the sheets. He used to take me to some lovely places, and I never once felt that I was his dirty secret; I quickly felt that I was the woman he wanted to be with, and I would make up every excuse in the book to get out of the house and away from Glenn to be with Faisal.

We went to fabulous restaurants, he was amazingly attentive and he always paid me compliments. I felt 10 feet tall when I was with him in those early days. He treated me like I was a princess. And he showered me with gifts, like most Arabs do when they are first getting to know you. As far as I was concerned, this was a wonderful man who wanted to be with me and who wanted to show me off.

This wasn't a five-minute wonder. We had been having our affair for about a year and one day we were in a hotel room and I realised that it was my wedding anniversary. I have no idea whether or not Glenn knew that I was seeing somebody else, or whether he just chose to turn a blind eye to it. My feeling was that he was scared to ask if there was somebody else because he knew that I would tell him the truth. It is entirely possible, of course, that he hadn't a clue.

Anyway, I told Faisal that I needed to phone my husband, so there I was, lying in bed with my lover while wishing Glenn a happy anniversary. "Sorry I haven't phoned you earlier darling but you know what it's like when I go out with the girls – we all have a few drinks and then we just lose all track of time."

"Did you have a good time last night then?"

"Yes, it was all right, but I be home by midday and then we can spend the rest of the day together and do something nice."

"Okay, see you later Sarah."

During that period, every time I opened my mouth to speak to Glenn it seemed that I was telling him a pack of lies. "I am just going out tonight with a couple of girlfriends," but I didn't really have any girlfriends, and poor Glenn would never ask for details. He never wanted to know who or where.

Faisal announced that he was going to leave his wife, a woman he had already split up from once before, because he had fallen in love with me and wanted to spend the rest of his life with me. We had a long talk and I agreed that I would also leave Glenn. Faisal fulfilled his side of the deal straight away, but I kept putting it off. The fact of the matter was that I didn't want to hurt Glenn – here was a man who had shown me and my daughter nothing but love and kindness, and I was repaying him by having an affair behind his back. I felt like a heel.

I kept making excuses to Faisal. He was rapidly running out of patience with me and threatened to turn up at our house, tell Glenn what was happening and drag me out with him, and I was more than a little bit concerned that he might actually do it. I was terrified of making another mistake. Yes, we were having a great time together while we were having an affair, but I had been down that road before. Faisal was dangerous and exciting, and in the back of my mind I was worried that when we started to live together it might all go pear-shaped.

This time I was also determined that Charlotte would not suffer. I had to put her first, and I had to be certain that Faisal would accept her into his life and would treat her well. As it would turn out, he would become the stepfather from hell...

He used to phone me at home when he knew Glenn would be in, and I would have to pretend that I was talking to a girlfriend. To make matters worse, the Barracuda club was taken over and the new owners decided that there were too many staff, and I was told that my services were no longer required. It was around that time that Michael Rutt was released from prison and I helped him out with his Paramount escort agency.

Faisal found out what I was doing and told me that me didn't want me within a million miles of Rutt; he even said that he would pay me if I kept away. I agreed that I would cut my ties with Michael, but Faisal didn't realise I was still sneaking off to see him, so I was getting paid by Michael as well.

And there was the night of October 28, 1989. It was his 34th birthday and it should have been a memorable one. It certainly turned out to be memorable, but for all the wrong reasons. It turned out to be a night that I will never forget until the day I die. He was living in a rented property in Enfield that belonged to one of his friends and we had arranged to meet there before going out to celebrate his birthday. I had promised him that I would stay the night with him, and I was really looking forward to a great evening.

He had bought theatre tickets and booked a table at an expensive restaurant, and it was all going to be fantastic. I duly told Glenn that I was going out with one of my fictitious girlfriends and that I probably wouldn't be home until the next morning, and off I went. I have seldom look forward to a night more than I did that one.

I turned up at his house in a short skirt, high heels and a nice top and when he opened the door, holding a glass of champagne, he looked at me in horror.

"What are dressed like that for?"

"What do you mean?"

"You can't go out dressed like that. You've got red lipstick on."

I couldn't believe what I was hearing. I had dressed to please him. All of a sudden, the man who had loved to go out with me while I was wearing short skirts and sporting red lipstick had decided that he didn't like this anymore.

"Well I'm not changing."

"Take that lipstick off."

"I'm not taking it off."

"Take that fucking lipstick off."

Suddenly I was being subjected to a side of this man that I had never seen before. Some women – most women – would have backed off, but that wasn't my style. This was the way I dressed, and this was the way I looked. It had always been good enough for him before, so why not now?

We started to have a drink together, trying to defuse the situation. I said to him: "Come on Faisal, it's your birthday, let's try and have a nice time here."

I told him again that I wasn't going to change – even if I had wanted to, I didn't have anything else suitable for going out in. By now, we were in the lounge, and I was hopeful that we could rescue the evening, but there was no chance.

I believe he'd already had a drink or two before I arrived, and there was a look in his eye that left me deeply unsettled, and then he announced: "Well, I'm not going out with you while you are dressed like that, and that's an end to it. You'll have to go and get changed."

"I can't get changed. I haven't brought anything I can change into. I didn't realise you were suddenly going to become so unreasonable about my appearance. What do you want me to wear? It's eight o'clock in the evening – I can't go and buy anything. What do you want me to do?"

"Well I want you to take that lipstick off for a start." He had already smeared it across my face. I was resigned to the fact that we weren't going out anywhere, so I put my glass down, deciding that I was going to head home to Glenn.

I threw my arms in the air and said: "Obviously we are not going anywhere tonight. Fine. I am going, I'm out of here."

I started walking towards the door and all of a sudden what felt like a brick crashed into the back of my head. It had been his fist, and I fell to the floor. He had knocked me senseless with that single blow. I hadn't a clue what had happened to me; I just couldn't connect with the fact that this man whom I loved had struck me. It was like I had been shot.

But that was only the start of it. The next thing I knew, he was dragging me by my hair up the spiral staircase. At the top of the stairs was the bedroom, and he pulled me in there, slammed the door shut and smashed my face into the door handle. There was blood everywhere, and I knew that I was in serious trouble.

It entered my mind that I was going to die, right there, right then.

He threw me on the bed and then he started ripping my clothes off and raped me. He was like a wild animal, and his eyes were dead, devoid of feeling and emotion. He kept repeating: "This is what you deserve, you bitch. Whore, tart, slag..."

He then turned me over and raped me from behind, and all the while he kept punching my face. I remember trying to reach for the phone, which was on a bedside table, but he pulled it from my hand and threw it across the room.

I wanted it all to be over, but he was just getting into his stride. He repeatedly spat at me, sank his teeth into various parts of my flesh and scratched me. It was exactly like being attacked by a lion or a tiger that is about to kill its prey.

When, finally, it was all over, he stood up and said: "Well that's exactly what you deserve. Now we are definitely not going out for dinner, are we?"

I was in a state of shock. There was blood pouring from various injuries on my head and face, and I was also bleeding down below. Every part of my body hurt, but I knew that, somehow, I had to find a way to get out of the house, so I did the only thing that I thought would work, and I apologised to him. I knew that he had taken leave of his senses, probably fuelled by drink, but I also knew that I had to let him continue to feel that he was in control, that what he had done was entirely normal and that he had nothing to reproach himself about.

By now, he was sitting down, smoking a cigarette. He had a bottle of whisky in one hand and was drinking straight from it. A survival instinct kicked in and I heard myself apologising to him. "I hope you enjoyed that, you slag." I just agreed, and tried to pick up my clothes, or what was left of them, and get dressed.

I was pretty certain that he had broken my legs but I somehow managed to get myself dressed, all the while thinking: "Don't antagonise him, don't antagonise him. You have just got to get out of here and get yourself home."

I picked up my bag and managed to get to the bedroom door, with the stairs he had dragged me up directly in front of me. I could sense that Faisal was behind me, but I couldn't hear properly because there was a buzzing in my ears. As I got to the top of the stairs he kicked me in the back and I fell, and tumbled all the way to the bottom. I don't know how I survived, but still it wasn't over.

As I lay on the floor, he came running down the stairs after me and jumped on my face. He then knelt over me, started punching me and spitting in my face again and then he held my face in his hands and said: "Why don't you die? You should be dead. I want you to die." He repeated this, over and over again.

He then went into the kitchen and as I lay there I could only imagine what new horror he was about to inflict upon me. When he returned, he had a pair of scissors, which he duly used to hack off all my hair.

The punches continued to rain down on me, mostly focused upon my face. He had knocked a couple of my teeth out and chipped most of the others. My cheekbones were broken, as was my jaw and my eye sockets. This man that I loved, this man I would have done anything for, had set out to destroy the way I looked – and all because the skirt I had chosen to wear had been too short, and the lipstick I had applied was not a colour he liked on that particular night.

Still my ordeal wasn't over. "Why aren't you dead? You should be dead." With that, he jumped on me again, this time puncturing one of my lungs.

And, finally, it was over. Satisfied with his night's work, he suddenly got to his feet and, without a word, went into the lounge and sat down, leaving me motionless on the floor, with blood everywhere.

I had been drifting in and out of consciousness throughout, and my eyes were so badly bruised that I was struggling to see anything, but at one point I looked back up the stairs and saw so much blood spattered everywhere that I recall thinking that it was just like a scene from the film *The Texas Chainsaw Massacre*.

It was like a murder scene. My murder scene. Only somehow I wasn't dead. I still had the presence of mind to keep thinking that I had to get out because it was obvious that he wasn't going to do anything to help me; indeed, he could start his attack on me again at any second.

I then started to vomit as I was choking on my own blood. Just thinking about it all these years later is a deeply upsetting experience. I would never have believed that jealousy, because that's what it was, could fuel such evil and wickedness in a person who was supposed to love and care for me.

Despite the state I was in, I had sufficient presence of mind to know that if I didn't get out, and soon, then he would get his wish and I would be dead. Every time I tried to say something to him, he simply replied: "I am waiting for you to die bitch. Just fucking die will you. I want you to die."

My bag was lying next to me, and inside it were my car keys. I could see the front door and the balcony beyond it, and I knew that I somehow had to drag myself to the door and get to my car, but because he had punctured my lung, even the very act of trying to draw breath was sheer agony. I had to summon up all my strength to get away. I just had to.

Charlotte's image popped into my head. "I've got to get out, I've got to get out. I must find a way. I must find a way. I don't want to lie here and give that bastard the satisfaction of watching me die. Fight it Sarah, fight it. I've got to get out."

With all the strength that I could muster, I managed to get myself upright and grab hold of the banister. Faisal had drunk so much by this

95

point that he was just about passed out on the chair, so I threw myself at the door and somehow managed to get it open. When I got outside I screamed as loudly as I could. There were flats everywhere, but nobody came to help me. Not one single person lifted a finger, or even came to their front door to find out what was going on.

To get to my car I had to get down another flight of stairs and I knew that the only way I could get down them was by allowing myself to fall down, and that's what I did. I was in so much pain that it hardly seemed to matter what additional damage I did to myself. Besides, the adrenalin had kicked in by now. I belief we all possess a sense of self-preservation and I had come this far and had no intentions of failing now.

It was very dark, and there was nobody about. As I reached my car and opened the door, he was behind me. He took my head in his hands and smashed it into the car door, and then closed the door on my hand, breaking my fingers.

I was half in and half out of my car and he hauled me out and started his assault all over again. He punched me again and again and again. By now, I felt nothing. This was what it felt like just before you die. He finally stopped when he caught sight of two people walking not far away, and then he bent down and pretended to kiss me.

I was like a rag doll. When the couple walked by, Faisal let me go, turned away and went back up the stairs. I fell to the floor, my face utterly destroyed.

My survival instinct got me into my car and I somehow managed to drive it to the nearest police station. I then staggered out, tumbled into the police station and collapsed on the floor, utterly spent. The attack on me was recorded at Enfield police station as Major Crime 2831, and it was timed at 1.30am.

CHAPTER 11
Sins Of The Father

I woke up in hospital, but they would not operate on me because they knew that they were dealing with a rape case, which meant that I had to be subjected to a full medical examination and police interview. I was designated a case officer, a WPC Fitzgerald, who not only interviewed me, but counselled me at great length about what I had been through. She was horrified at the extent of my injuries and couldn't believe they had been inflicted by somebody who professed to love me. She would eventually refer me to the victim support programme, but I decided to deal with things my own way.

I was swabbed, poked and prodded. It was a dreadful experience. I overheard a doctor saying: "We have got to get this right. All the tests need to be done properly because we have got to do everything we can to help the police find the man who did this."

"I know who did it....."

Within hours, Faisal was in custody.

Eventually I came round properly and the first thing I wanted to do was to look at myself in a mirror. Fucking hell! I didn't know who that was, but it definitely wasn't me in the reflection. I looked like something out of a horror movie, and said to the nurse who was with me: "I wish that he had finished me off because he has destroyed me. Nobody will ever look at me in the same light again. I look like a freak show."

I could cope with all the other injuries, and even with the knowledge that the bastard had raped me, but I couldn't cope with what he had done to my looks. Everything I had managed to achieve up to that point in my life had been done as a result of the way I looked.

And that wasn't the end of the grief. You will remember that Glenn had thought I was going out with a friend.

The police had to knock on his door and tell him what had happened. I cannot begin to imagine what must have gone through his mind. "How could my wife possibly get beaten up and raped if she was out for the night with one of her friends?"

When he came to see me in hospital I was faced with two choices – I could either lie to him or I could finally tell him the truth, the thing that I am sure he had suspected for months anyway. I told him the truth. Glenn was amazing. He could have just turned on his heels and told me he wanted nothing more to do with me, and I couldn't possibly have blamed him if he had chosen that course of action. But he didn't. Instead, he wanted to go round and beat Faisal to a pulp, to do to him what he had done to me.

He didn't seemed too concerned about the fact that I'd been having an affair.

But I didn't tell my parents. I couldn't face telling them the truth.

I was in hospital for weeks and the National Health Service did its best to put me back together again, but they really weren't interested in whether my cheekbones were asymmetrical or whether my jaw looked right. They were worried about saving my life, and they did that. I have no issues with the way I was treated by the doctors and nurses.

As I got my strength back so my hatred for Faisal grew. I hated him, and I hated myself for what I had become and for what I had done to Glenn, and to Charlotte, who had to watch her Mum go through all this grief. Why couldn't I just have been happy with the hand I was dealt? Why couldn't I have settled for Glenn and the life he gave me?

When I was released from hospital Glenn was wonderful. There was never any question of him throwing me out. He welcomed me back into our home, but I was in the depths of depression. I couldn't bear to look at myself in the mirror and I started drinking in order to blot everything out.

My husband was incredibly kind and loving towards me, but then Faisal's wife started phoning me, begging me to drop the charges against him. On more than one occasion I did wonder what story he had spun her because surely, if she knew the truth, she would never have allowed him back across the threshold of her home. She told me that it would destroy him if he had to go to court. Destroy him? What about me?

But I listened, and she kept chipping away, until eventually she ground me down. My mind was made up. I went to see the police and told them I no longer wished to proceed, and that if the case went to court I would refuse to give evidence against him. They had no choice but to drop the charges. But for Glenn I suppose that was the final straw. If I could let a man who beat me to within an inch of my life walk free, then I guess Glenn must have figured that I still loved him, and there was no future for our marriage.

I look back on it now and I cannot believe the course of action I took. Faisal had a wife and daughter and I had put myself in their shoes and couldn't bear the thought of what might happen to them if it had gone to court. I was wrong. I should have seen it through. I should have seen him go to jail.

In an extraordinary twist to the tale, his daughter and mine would go on to become best friends, and I know that she does not think much of her father.

I no longer wanted to go out. All that I was interested in doing was sitting at home looking at the world through the bottom of a wine glass.

I had been a vibrant, sexually active woman, and now I was dead inside. It didn't help that I kept having nightmares about my attack – I sometimes think it might have been easier to deal with if it had been perpetrated by a total stranger. For somebody you love to violate you in such a shocking way takes some getting used to.

I felt ugly, that people were looking at me and were laughing and staring. For the first time in my life I felt self-conscious about my looks. I could not bear to see myself in a mirror. My self-confidence had been destroyed and I hated every part of my body. No matter what clothes I wore and no matter how hard I tried with make-up, nothing worked. I had become an ugly duckling.

I hated my hair, I hated my teeth, I hated my face. But the worst thing of all was that I knew that I could put it all right if I had money. I'd read all about plastic surgery and the various procedures that could be carried out, so I knew there was potential to rescue my looks. Sadly, the procedures I would need would cost many thousands of pounds, and I didn't have two pennies to rub together, and there was little or no prospect of that situation ever changing.

I couldn't go to a plastic surgeon and say: "Make me beautiful again." I had spoken to the NHS, but was told they had done everything they could for me. I was informed that I looked 'fine'. I didn't look 'fine' and even if I did, Sarah Goddard did not do 'fine'. Never had, never has, never will. Sarah Goddard only ever did beautiful.

I wanted my life back. The drink helped for a while because it deadened the pain, and I knew that I had to keep my act together sufficiently well to look after Charlotte, who now became the focus of my life. I made sure she got to school and that she was smartly dressed and clean, and I ensured that she was properly looked after. But who was going to look after me?

I would drop her off at school at 9am and then come straight home and start drinking. At 9am! By midday I would be on a different planet. I started to neglect myself and lost two stones in weight so I went to see my doctor.

His advice? "Pull yourself together."

"What do you mean, pull myself together?"

"I know you have had a dreadful experience Sarah, but it has also happened to other people. Maybe you need to talk to somebody."

"I don't need a psychiatrist. What I need is somebody who will put me back together again. I need a plastic surgeon."

"Stop being so vain."

"It is not about vanity. I have had everything taken away from me, everything that mattered, everything that I held most dear. So don't tell me that I am vain because I am not. I am just a woman who wants to get her old life and her old self back. It's really not too much to ask is it?"

Apparently it was.

Nobody deserved to be treated as I had been. It was like when the five women were murdered in Ipswich and every time I switched on the news I heard them referred to as prostitutes. They were women. First and foremost, they were women. Like me. I was a woman, a woman who had been beautiful and was now being accused of being vain because my looks had been taken away from me.

The doctor must have become sick of the sight of me because I kept going to see him and, of course, I would never admit that I was drinking copious amounts of alcohol, but I would hold my hand out and say: "Look, I am shaking, and I can't stop it." Well of course I was shaking – my system was full of booze.

I am ashamed to say that I twice tried to kill myself by popping a huge assortment of pills, and each time I ended up in hospital and had my stomach pumped. I was crying out for help but nobody was listening, or if they were then they weren't hearing what I was saying. Was I really trying to commit suicide, or was it a cry for help? I don't know.

The hospital staff thought I was an attention seeker, but they had no idea what had happened to me, and they would simply send me packing.

Back I went to the doctor, this time to complain about the pains I was feeling in my back and legs. Remember that not only had he subjected me to a savage beating, but he had also kicked me down a flight of stairs made of iron.

At my worst moment, I was sent to see a neurologist who listened as I told him about the various pains I was suffering. He conducted a series of tests and then dropped the latest bombshell to explode in my life. He told me that he was fairly certain I was suffering from multiple sclerosis. Could anything else go wrong? What was the point of carrying on?

I didn't know a huge amount about MS, but I knew enough to realise that it was degenerative and that it gradually attacked your body until you reached the stage where you couldn't walk. And I was told that I was going to have to take steroids as part of the treatment. Steroids – didn't they turn women into big fat blobs? And didn't they have 1,001 other potential side-effects, not one of them pleasant? I was utterly devastated.

I ended up back in hospital for a week while they devised the best course of treatment for me. There are different types of MS and they all respond in different ways to different drugs. I had some awful things done to me while I was in hospital, not least a lumbar-puncture and electric shock treatment.

At the end of it all the consultant came in to see me, and he had umpteen young trainee doctors with him. He had lots of papers in his hand – all the test results, I guess – and he said: "Mmmm, it's very difficult to diagnose MS, but yes, I think you've got it."

I asked him to explain what it meant it terms of how it might affect the rest of my life. "Well, in the worst-case scenario, you could be dead in five years," he replied. This verdict was delivered in a very matter-of-fact manner. To him I was just another number.

So I no longer had my looks, and now I might only have five years left to live.

As I prepared to leave, a nurse gave me lots of leaflets and various other bits and pieces that described MS and its assorted symptoms. She also told me that I would be able to claim various disability benefits, something that hadn't even entered my head.

I wanted to cut my throat. My head was spinning. Glenn and I were still together at this point, but that was the moment when I decided that I was going to move out and that we were going to go our separate ways. I didn't want some man clucking around me, looking after me, waiting on me hand and foot as I lived out the final months and years of my life. I knew that if nothing had been wrong with me then I would be moving out anyway, and as far as my marriage was concerned, this diagnosis made no difference at all, other than to confirm that I needed some space. Apart from anything else, I had already given this man far too much grief. He deserved better.

He couldn't understand my reasoning when I sat him down and told him that our marriage was over and that I was moving out. He genuinely did want to look after me – during the weeks and months when I was recovering from the attack, most men would have thrown my relationship with Faisal back in my face, but Glenn didn't.

He was a kind, compassionate and caring individual, but I didn't love him. I am not sure that I ever did. A number of strange things happened while I was with Glenn, including a phone call I received from Tony Burge, the boy I had met on holiday all those years earlier, when life seemed far less complicated.

He had contacted my mother and asked for my phone number, telling her he would love to get back in touch with me. Mum always liked Tony, so she gave him my number. I ended up meeting him and together we went to the premier of the James Bond movie, *The Living Daylights*, and we slept together.

Tony told me he had missed me and asked me to move in with him but I refused because, at the time, I was married to Glenn and was in the throes of my affair with Faisal.

One other huge complication occurred at this time. I discovered that I was pregnant, and I hadn't a clue who the father was. It could have been Glenn, it could have been Faisal, and it could even have been Tony. I know that I must sound like a right slapper and, once again, it was not something that filled me with pride. I couldn't bear the thought of bringing a child into the world and not knowing who was the father so my way of dealing with the problem was to go back to a clinic and have another abortion.

Having been down that road once before, it was not a pleasant experience to do it again, but it was made easier for me when Glenn found out I was pregnant and announced that he didn't want any children. "I don't want a baby, so you can get rid of it," he said. That meant that at least I was able to count on his support during what was a difficult time, although once again I suspected that perhaps the real reason he didn't want me to have it was because he knew I was having an affair and he suspected the child might not be his.

Faisal also knew that I was pregnant, and it was all threatening to become incredibly complicated. Having an abortion was the only way I could deal with it, and in the end it was Faisal who took me to the clinic. All the way there he kept pleading with me: "Don't get rid of it, don't get rid of it."

"But Faisal, I have already told you that I don't know whose baby it is."

"It doesn't matter whose baby it is. You can't get rid of it. You must not get rid of it. You are killing a human being. You are ending a life."

I was not in a good place, and this was the last thing I needed to be hearing.

And afterwards he refused to let the subject drop.

Nothing was ever simple in my life. But now I was rid of them all. I got myself a flat and moved in with Charlotte and although I signed on and claimed benefits, I drew the line at claiming disability benefit. I had no job, and I had no money. The lowest I ever felt was one day when I realised that I didn't have enough money to buy a pint of milk. Fortunately, I kept hold of a lot of the stuff from my Playboy days, so I gradually sold all the jewellery and all the flash clothes, apart from a fur coat that I made up my mind I was going to keep.

Funnily enough, I always managed to scrape together the money to buy booze. It was my escape. Eventually I woke up to the fact that if I carried on drinking every day then it was probably going to kill me, but how I didn't become a crazed alcoholic I will never know.

With my life in tatters, I decided to turn to religion and started attend my local church. To be honest, I didn't expect that it would help or that it would give me any comfort but it did, in the most unexpected way.

I know that I might seem a pretty unlikely candidate for religion, but I was dying, and the first thing anybody does in that situation is to run to God. I had read about it, and I had seen it in trashy films, so I thought: "Why not? It might even help me."

First of all I made up my mind that Charlotte was going to be christened, so I arranged to see the vicar, explained my circumstances and yes, of course he was only too happy to open the doors of his church to me.

The vicar's name was Peter, and he was a very good listener. It felt good to speak to somebody that I didn't know, and talking about what I had been through did help me. I ended up telling him my life story and rather than judging me, he listened. He just listened. It was such a refreshing change not to have somebody telling me I should have done this, or I should be doing that.

Surprisingly, I threw myself into church life and I realised that I no longer needed to drink to get through the day. Apart from Peter, I began to form a relationship with some of the other parishioners, and many of them would come and visit Charlotte and I at our flat. Like Peter, they did not judge me either. They all knew my story, knew what I had been through, but accepted me for what I was, warts and all.

Suddenly, I had a brand new circle of friends, and I was going to church every Sunday – what's more, I used to look forward to the services, and to hearing what Peter had to say. And apart from services, I used to go there once or twice a day, every day, because I was able to find some comfort. I am not going to pretend that I had found God, or that I had seen the light, but there was definitely something. Maybe it felt good because I was at a stage in my life where I needed something.

For the first time in my life I had women friends, and I found that difficult to come to terms with. In the past, women had always steered clear of me because they saw me as a threat. Now I found myself wondering: "Are these women happy to be in my company because I am ugly and boring now? Why is it that suddenly everybody seems to like me? Is it because I am becoming a real person inside? Or is it because I am going to die and they feel pity for me?"

Peter lived in a house not far from the church and I used to visit him there. At first, it was all perfectly innocent, but I realised that I was attracted to him as a man, and one thing led to another. Before I knew where I was, the two of us were have an affair. We made love at the vicarage on a regular basis, and I am ashamed to admit that we even made love in the church. May God forgive me.

In truth, I think he was bored and was looking for a bit of excitement, and I was happy to provide him with it. Our relationship lasted for a few weeks and one day I turned up for a service and Peter wasn't there. The church had sent along a replacement.

Afterwards, one of the women came over to me and when I asked where Peter was she replied: "Haven't you heard Sarah? He has been diagnosed with multiple sclerosis. Can you believe it?"

No, I couldn't believe it. This was the cruellest twist of fate. Somebody up there really didn't like me. I had found a small crumb of comfort, something to take my mind off my own illness and everything else that was going on in my life, and now I was being told that Peter had MS. It was too much.

At this point I should probably explain that I lived every day as if it were my last. I wasn't sure when I was going to start getting spasms, and when I was going to end up in a wheelchair, utterly dependent upon somebody else to look after even my most basic requirements.

But nothing was happening to me. Apart from the depression that I felt, physically I did not seem to be deteriorating in any way, so I kept going back to the doctor and asking why, and he kept fobbing me off. His attitude was that if the top man in the field had told me that I had multiple sclerosis, then there was not the slightest doubt in his mind that I did have it.

Only I didn't. It would emerge years later that all the mental turmoil I had been put through was for nothing. Not only that, but I discovered that it would never leave me because it was on my medical records – if I wanted to get a job in a casino and they wanted to check my medical history, there it would be in black and white. And the fact that the diagnosis was wrong, would make no difference. I was tainted for life, and all because a specialist had made a mistake.

Sadly, the same could not be said for Peter. His diagnosis was correct and the deterioration in his health was fairly swift. He could not continue with his duties, was moved by the church and the two of us lost touch with one another.

CHAPTER 12
In Bed With The Devil

About a year had passed since Faisal's attack. The vicar had come and gone and I had decided that the church was not for me after all. Perhaps Peter had been the attraction all along.

Charlotte and I were still living in the flat and I wish I could say that we were living happily ever after, but we weren't. In truth, I was going downhill fairly rapidly. I looked and felt worn-out.

My relationship with my mother was very uneasy. She couldn't understand the way I had been able to go from one man to another, from one relationship straight into another, from one commitment to another. This was my hour of need, and I should have been able to go to my Mum and Dad, but I felt that I had nobody. I also managed to convince myself that I didn't need anybody. Obviously, that was rubbish. I needed help and support at that time more than any other in my life.

I could never talk to my mother and explain how I felt. Earlier, I wrote about the way she liked to brush things under the carpet. It's not her fault; that was the way she was brought up. Her generation were taught that it was best not to confront things head on, but to sidestep them. That way, they would simply go away.

And she couldn't get to grips with the fact that we were living in a very different sort of society. I wasn't alone in jumping from one relationship to another. Lots of people did it, men and women. When Mum got married, it was expected to be for life.

Personally, I could imagine nothing worse than living with a man I did not love, and that is perhaps why I have had too many relationships; there were times when maybe I should have stayed and tried to work things out, but my problem was that I was impetuous. I did things without ever thinking about the consequences. I married John because I thought that I loved him. I married Glenn because I thought he was an exciting artist, but he turned out to be somebody with whom I nothing in common. And I got involved with Faisal because he was a charismatic Arab who treated me the way I wanted to be treated. Right up until the point where he turned his fists and his feet on me.

Things started to look up for me when I managed to get a job back at the Barracuda club, and because I had worked for the company in the past, there was no need for a medical. But I had to confront one major problem. Faisal worked there.

From day one, he tried to worm his way back into my life and my affections. Although he'd got his wife to do his dirty work by phoning me up and pleading with me to get the charges dropped, he wasn't living with her. He had his own place, and he quickly made it clear that he wanted me back.

"I know I have done wrong, and I hate to see you like this. I should be looking after you, taking care of you. I should be making sure that you want for nothing, that you are fit and well and healthy," he said.

He came round to my flat and said he was horrified at the conditions in which I was living. "You don't have to live like this Sarah," he said. "Come and live with me, you and Charlotte. It will be good between us. We can be together and I will look after Charlotte. And I promise that I will never do anything like that ever again."

I believed him, and so it was that I moved myself and my daughter into his home. I know that many of you will think that I was completely insane, but I truly felt that I had no other option. I had little or no money – if I went to live with him, he would pay all the bills and I could start to save some cash. Besides, if you have learnt anything at all about me, you will know that I am not a person who could live without a man in my life.

Yes, I was wary of him. Very wary indeed. But at this point in my life I still believed that I was dying from MS, and I wanted to enjoy some comfort. You can have no idea what it feels like to be told that you could be dead within five years until you have heard those words for yourself – and I hope that nobody who reads this will ever have to endure that.

I had tried to kill myself because I figured that I could do it on my own terms. The thought of being pushed around in a wheelchair filled me with horror.

I needed an easy way out, and I needed somebody to look after me. Faisal was genuinely sorry for what he had done. It didn't make it right, and it didn't mean that I forgave him. How could I? Every morning I got up, looked in the bathroom mirror and was reminded of what this man had done to me. And now I was back in his bed.

Was I completely mad? I am happy to let you be the judge of that for yourself.

I got involved with the MS Society, doing a lot of voluntary work for them. And I caught a glimpse of what my future would be like when I used to help some of the sufferers to write their letters because they could no longer do so themselves. And I would take them to the hospital for their appointments because I was the only one who could walk unaided.

This was one thing that I had shared with both my parents and with Trevor, my brother, who by now was in America. He started looking into what treatments might be available in the United States, where they also seeming to be developing pioneering drugs. Every time we got together, we all ended up in tears – me, my Mum and my Dad.

After a while, Faisal and I bought a house in Pinner, which was an area I had always liked. Everything was all right at first, and he was the man who had originally wooed me, but it didn't take long for things to change. He turned into a complete and utter bastard. He was a bully, verbally and physically.

He had his good days, of course, but usually I couldn't do anything right for him. And that is when I knew that I needed a long-term plan. I decided to make the most of it and stick it out for as long as I could; in the meantime, every penny that I could get my hands on was being squirrelled away.

I decided that I would use him in any way that I could, and ended up living a lie for the best part of ten years in order to get out of the mess I was in. I was determined that I would get my looks sorted out, that I would look after my health and that I would do the best I possibly could for Charlotte. Yes, I could have walked out on him and gone straight back into another flat and signed up for benefits again, but where would that have got me?

Gradually, I learnt how to read his moods, and knew what to do and what to say to achieve self-preservation. I should have got out, I know that now.

Most of my life was spent treading on egg-shells. We had to be particularly careful in the morning because we never knew what mood he was going to be in when he woke up. But for all the abuse he used to hurl at me, it was the way he spoke to Charlotte that used to make my skin crawl.

He treated her and spoke to her like she was something he had stepped in. It makes me want to weep when I think about it now. He verbally abused her so badly that she would go to her room and stay there all day. She didn't want to come out, and she didn't want to mix with friends, and all because he destroyed her self-confidence. And every time he spoke to her that way, or raised his voice to her, I would step in so that he could use me as his verbal (and physical) punch-bag.

Through that period, Charlotte and I grew closer together, I suppose because I felt the way a lioness does when she is protecting her cubs – she doesn't want anything to happen to them. We were more than mother and daughter – we were best friends too.

I make no bones about it – there were times when I would look at him and murderous thoughts would go through my mind, but I was determined not to stoop to his level.

Besides, there was my escape plan. I didn't know whether I was ever going to be able to pull it off, but I was determined that I was going to give it my best shot, When I left this relationship, it was going to be on my terms, not his.

He worked nights and slept through most of the day, so we didn't have to spend huge amounts of time in his company, but I should never have put Charlotte through it, especially as it came on top of all the other traumas that she had been through.

I felt that I had no option, that I had no nobody to turn to for help. People will judge me, I know they will, and will almost certainly come to the conclusion that I have been a bad mother, but until anybody has walked a hundred miles in my shoes I defy them to decry me. I was just trying to survive.

Lots of women get involved in abusive relationships and people ask why they stay, why they don't walk away, but it is seldom as simple as that. There are more options now than there were back then, that's for sure, but for many women even today it takes huge amounts of courage to pick yourself up, pack your worldly goods into a case or bin bag and throw yourself on the mercy of a women's refuge or, if you are very, very lucky, a loving relative.

He regularly hit me, and seemed to take great delight in kicking me. Inevitably, he kicked me down a flight of stairs when I was pregnant with his daughter. What sort of a man does that? Remember that this was the man who pleaded with me not to have the abortion. And now, when he knew that I was pregnant with his child, he thought it was all right to use my body for target practice, or to use me as a punch bag.

Although the attacks were fairly frequent, they never again came close to the intensity or ferocity of the first one, and I made up my mind that I could cope with it. Maybe he wanted me to beg him to stop, but I was never going to give him that satisfaction. He would hit me and I would try to show no emotion, but I always ended up fighting back like a wild cat.

What used to set him off? He hated it if I didn't load the dishwasher properly, or if I left something in the sink. Or if there was no top on the toothpaste tube, and the toothpaste was coming out of the tube – he would go absolutely mental. Like a raging bull.

I couldn't cook (and still can't), and that could have caused conflict too, but he accepted that at the outset. In any event, he enjoyed cooking, just as long as I was the one who cleaned up his mess after him.

The hardest thing for me to deal with was that everybody who met Faisal was charmed by him because he could really turn on the style. He had women eating out of the palm of his hand, and he was able to hold his own with men on most subjects.

"Oh Sarah, he is so lovely, you are so lucky to have him," my friends would say. And the minute they had left our house I would get a slap because of some innocent remark I had made during the night; something he would have stewed about until he got the chance to get it out of his system. Most normal human beings would sit their partner down and say: "I wish you hadn't said that earlier," and would then go on to explain why they felt the way they did. With Faisal it was just easier to hit me.

If the next door neighbour was struggling to, say, put up a fence, Faisal would be the first in the queue, offering to help, so they also thought he was a wonderful man. They didn't know about the tears I wept almost every night of my life over the way he treated me.

I had switched off emotionally. It was the only way I could get through it.

Then I decided that I wanted to do something to improve my lot and made up my mind that I was going to go to college and learn to become a beautician. He wasn't happy about it, and I had to give him more sex to pacify him, but I was determined that he wasn't going to stand in my way. It was another part of the escape plan.

This turned out to be the most difficult thing I had ever done. I was working nights at the Barracuda, then I was at college during the day and then there was the pregnancy, something that wasn't planned. For a while, I was walking around like a zombie. I used to fantasise about being able to go to bed and go to sleep, but I was driven on by the thought of getting a qualification, moving out and going on to build a better life for me and my family.

I was overjoyed when my second daughter was born. Hannah would grow up to hate and despise her father. Not long after she was born, Faisal said something to me that brought home to me just what a monster I was living with. The baby was crying and he said: "She's being naughty. Why don't you wallop her?"

I could just about live with what he had done to me over the years, but the thought that he could ever treat his own child in such a way stopped me in my tracks. I looked at him and said: "Wallop her? She is a tiny baby. I will wallop you in a minute – and don't you ever raise a finger to her."

By now, I was regularly having visions of killing him in his sleep, and given the right set of circumstances, it is something I might easily have done. I fantasised about getting a kitchen knife and slashing his throat, and on more than one occasion I actually went into the kitchen and picked up a suitable knife. Thank God it never went past the point of being a sick fantasy.

When he raised his voice to the children it was like a red rag to a bull as far as I was concerned, and I would leave him in no doubt whatsoever about how I felt about him shouting at them. I used to tell him to pick on somebody his own size, and that was usually the signal for him to punch or kick me. Better that than he hit the kids though.

If I ever thought that he was about to raise his hand to them, I would throw myself at him. This was not a loving relationship. "If you ever hit my girls I will get a knife and I will stab you, and if I don't finish you off there and then, I will come to the hospital and I will cut off you life support system," I would scream at him.

When Hannah was born, we bought a dog called Pebbles for Charlotte – mainly because I wanted Charlotte to know how important she was to me, and believed it was vital that she didn't feel left out. In the end, I had to get rid of the poor animal because Faisal used to kick it and throw it against the wall. It was like it gave him some sort of cheap thrill, and it was pathetic, but this was a living creature, and I couldn't bear to watch it being treated in this way. Needless to say, Charlotte was distraught when I gave Pebbles away, but I was convinced that if I hadn't done so then he would have killed it.

Some of the waitresses at the Barracuda knew what the real Faisal was like because I would confide in them. I had to tell somebody what I was being subjected to back at home. At first they found it hard to believe but I then they would see little signs, times where he would be struggling to keep it together in company, and they would know I was telling them the truth. I was offered rooms in people's houses, as some of the girls told me that I had to get away from him, but my answer was always the same: I knew what I was doing, and I would be fine.

By now I was also working as a waitress, which meant that I didn't have to spend each night at work in his company. Faisal, remember, worked in the reception area. I even took my life in my hands by going out with other men behind his back. I needed to prove to myself that I was still attractive to men, despite what he had done to me. And, frankly, I needed some love. I wanted to feel wanted. I needed to be desired. These were normal emotions and feelings.

At one point I had an affair with a man called David Campbell, who told me that his mother was a duchess and who claimed to be part of the family who owned the renowned soup company. Although he was very wealthy, for all that I know, he may well have been spinning me a line, but it is one of the regrets of my life that when he asked me to leave Faisal I refused to do so. Even now, I am not sure why I said no.

I learnt to speak a bit of Arabic because I remembered that when I was throwing my well-worn Chinese phrases around all those years before it resulted in bigger and better tips than the rest of the girls were earning. Many of the customers at the Barracuda were Arabs and, sure enough, they loved it when somebody made an effort to speak to them in their own tongue. And it was once again reflected in the size of the tips I was receiving.

An added bonus of this was that when Faisal tried to belittle me in front of his mates, I could tell him to 'Fuck off' in Arabic. He hated that.

Despite everything I had been through at Italia Conti, I put Charlotte through stage school because it was her passion. She received a scholarship, but I had to make up the difference, which was no easy task for a waitress. I needed to make Faisal think it was a real struggle, and that I had no money left. That wasn't true though. By now, I had several thousand pounds in my escape fund, a bank account that he knew nothing about. Still not quite enough to give me my freedom, but I was getting there. If he knew I had that money, he would have taken it. There is no doubt in my mind. And I dread to think what he would have done to me.

Faisal was particularly beastly to Charlotte whenever his own daughter, Veronica, came round to see us. It was almost as if he did it because he wanted Veronica to know that he favoured her over my daughter. Veronica would later comment on it. "Charlotte, he was always so awful to you. I couldn't believe the way he spoke to you, the things he used to say to you," she would say in later years. It took a long time before Veronica felt able to make her own peace with her father.

Oh yes, and he would also take great delight in my plight. He would bang the worktop and say stuff like: "You're so fucking thick, but never mind because you are going to be dead soon, you fucking cripple." This was the man who claimed to love me.

Throughout my life when I have set out to get from A to B, I have always worked out what I needed to do to reach my destination. This was all about accumulating enough money, and when I felt that I had done that, then I could get to B, leaving Faisal and everything he stood for, far, far behind me.

I needed to repair myself and, here was the key, I need to complete my education. For me, completing my education meant finishing the course that would allow me to call myself a qualified beautician. I had made half-hearted attempts at various things throughout my life, but I was serious about this goal because I realised how much money there was to be made in the beauty industry – if you have any doubts about what I am saying, just take a walk along any High Street in any town or city and see how many hair and beauty salons there are.

It seemed ironic to me that after dreaming my way through mainstream education and then drama school, I had now finally realised the importance of getting a qualification. I was an ageing waitress with fading looks, and if I didn't come up with a contingency plan I was going to end up on benefits for the rest of my life because nobody would employ me – or at least nobody who was prepared to offer a decent salary would employ me.

I didn't want to end up living in a council house again.

First of all I learnt all about nails, everything I needed to know to become a manicurist. Next, I focused on beauty therapy, where you learn about bones and arteries and God-alone knows what else. Let's just say that it was slightly more complicated than learning to look after people's nails, but nothing that is worthwhile in life ever comes easy.

I did some of it at college, and paid to learn some parts of the job privately, purely and simply because it was easier to do things that way. Apart from anything else, if I had followed through on the college course it would have taken me three years to get the qualification I needed, but by doing it privately I was able to cram it into six months.

By this time in my life, I was just about reaching the end of my tether with Faisal, and didn't know how much longer I could stand being under the same roof as him.

Surprisingly, I found it incredibly easy to absorb all the knowledge that was being thrown at me – I suppose because I had the correct mindset. For once in my life, my mind was open to the things I was being taught and shown, and I became like a sponge, simply soaking it all up. It was wonderful.

The more they threw at me, the more I learnt. And the more I learnt, the hungrier I became for even more. If I had been able to treat school in this way, who knows what I might have achieved? In saying that, I was not being taught by sadistic nuns – I was being taught by normal human beings, whose only goal in life was to make sure that their message was getting across to the people who sat in front of them.

I was interested in what I was taught, and I guess that made it easier to absorb it all.

Then I found myself doing a course on semi-permanent make-up, and I learnt how to treat burns victims and to camouflage facial injuries – this was proper stuff, and it was meaningful. I learnt how to disguise facial scars and what make-up could be used to cover various types of skin conditions.

Faisal didn't fully understand what I was doing and that was great because it meant he wasn't especially interested, so he just let me get on with it. As long as the house was clean and I was there to have sex with him when he demanded it, life was just about bearable. I got through it all because I knew that there was soon going to be a way out for me, and that thought kept me going.

As I raced through all these courses and passed the exams and picked up the certificates, I made up my mind that I didn't want to go and work in some salon. I needed to be in Harley Street, working alongside the plastic surgeons – not just any old plastic surgeons, but the men who were the very best in the business. I figured that I could provide a com-plementary service, so a patient would go a see a top plastic surgeon, have whatever treatment they wanted, and then I could offer my services afterwards.

To me, it all made perfect sense. It didn't turn out to be quite as simple as that. I ended up pounding the pavements of Harley Street for months, knocking on doors, making appointments to speak to the surgeons, telling them what I could do, offering to assist them with post-operative care. With a breast augmentation, there would be scars, and I had the knowledge and the skills to be able to hide those scars.

Nobody was interested. Had I really gone through all of this for nothing? It would have been all too easy to have given up, but that wasn't my style. It never had been, and it certainly was going to be now, not if I wanted to get away from this man who was killing me inside. I felt that the longer I stayed with Faisal that as each day passed, so another tiny piece of me would die.

I realised that several Arab doctors used the casino and I ended up arranging to go out to dinner with them. Perhaps this was going to be my big break. But no, because it soon emerged that although they would go through the motions of listening to my pitch, all they really wanted to do was get me into bed.

It was hugely frustrating. Nobody seemed to be prepared to take me seriously, but I knew that I was on to something.

Eventually somebody did give me a chance, and I ended up working at 134 Harley Street. The deal was that I rented a room and advertised my services in various magazines. As I gained in confidence and started to build a client base, I began to learn about skin peeling and laser treatment and attended various courses in order to gain the relevant qualifications to perform those procedures.

It was all a case of 'you scratch my back and I will scratch yours', and as I began to stock and use certain products, so the manufacturers of those products would start putting customers my way.

By this stage, I had some money, and I quickly found out which doctors specialised in which areas of expertise, so I decided that the time had come to have my face put back together again.

CHAPTER 13
We Can Rebuild You

I started knocking on the doors of plastic surgeons in Harley Street all over again, but this time I had something to offer them.

"I have customers I am treating and they are looking for referrals, but they haven't the foggiest idea who they can trust and who they can't, and they are asking me who I would recommend," I explained. "I am not a particularly great advert at the moment, but I could be, and I have an idea that I would like you to consider..."

My idea was that they would perform various procedures on my face and I would become their walking advertisement. A human guinea pig, if you like.

You want a nose job? Here, look at what Mr X did for me. You need a new jawline? Here, take a look – Mr A is the man you want.

The problem was that these men could not advertise their services back then, and certainly not in the way that I was offering. Back then it was all word of mouth, and that meant if you were trying to establish yourself as a cosmetic surgeon then it could be a real struggle because you had nobody to vouch for what you could do. Let's face it, if you are going to spend a huge amount of money on a facelift, you want to be 100% certain that the man who is going to perform it knows exactly what he is doing because the last thing on earth that any of us want is to have the bandages removed and discover that we look like the bride of Frankenstein because the surgeon has learnt his skills through a correspondence course.

As far as I was concerned, what I was offering seemed like a win-win situation for everybody.

And so my journey into plastic surgery began. Initially, the surgeon would give me a small discount, but the more people I referred, the bigger the discount became for my next procedure. Bit by bit, I had everything repaired and had my face put back together. And then I got totally carried away.

During this time, I became quite a high-profile individual in and around Harley Street, and my name was being bandied about by a lot of doctors. I was using a skin peel product called Glyderm – as far as I was concerned, it was tried and tested and it worked. It came with a daily maintenance programme that featured a cream and moisturiser which the customer would apply themselves.

It wasn't rocket science – none of the products used in beauty therapy are particularly complicated. Much of it is just a matter of common sense. Anyway, this stuff exfoliated the skin. I was happy to use it on my own skin, as well as on the skin of my clients, and that was always one of my golden rules – I would never use anything on a customer that I hadn't tried myself first of all.

GM-TV used to have a feature called The Beauty Trap, fronted by Fiona Phillips, where they would send in an undercover reporter to Harley Street to try out various products – it was designed to stamp out sharp practice, and I thought that it was a good idea. They would basically expose products that didn't deliver, or focus on potions and lotions that customers were being charged exorbitant amounts of money for by unscrupulous individuals.

They were especially hard-hitting on products that they felt were overpriced and I am sure you have already guessed that they singled out

Glyderm. It wasn't a cheap product, but then again, it wasn't cheap for people like myself to buy in the first place, and, like every other business, I had to make some kind of a profit. I wasn't a charity, after all.

As far as I was concerned, the woman sitting in front of me was just another customer, who had come along with somebody who had severe acne. In fact, she turned out to be an undercover reporter called Carla Romano. The manufacturers of Glyderm recommended their product as a treatment for acne sufferers – I want to make it perfectly clear that at no stage did the manufacturer, or yours truly, ever claim that Glyderm would cure acne. There is no cure. But it would ease the condition.

There was something about this woman's acne that didn't ring true. Don't forget that I have a stage background and I had studied all sorts of beauty treatments. I looked at her and knew that something wasn't right, and if I'd had my wits about me, I would have shown them both the door.

She asked me: "Are you saying that Glyderm treats acne?"

Of course she wanted me to say yes, that it did, but what I actually said was: "You may or may not have acne, but this product can help control acne. And it can help your skin."

She then looked me up and down and asked: "Are those breasts real?"

She was clearly trying to get me at my ease, and I was able to tell her that yes, they were real.

The other woman then asked me about Glyderm once again. "So does it treat acne?"

This had been going on for sometime, and she had finally ground me down. "Yes, if that's what you want to hear, it treats acne."

They had what they wanted. The women had hidden cameras and, as is the way with these things, they were able to go away with their film, put it through an editing suite and totally distort the conversation that had taken place, and managed to make it look as if I was making false promises for Glyderm.

Two days later I got a phone called from the producers to tell me that they had sent undercover reporters into my office and that what they had managed to get on film would be shown on the Friday of that week on GM-TV. I was stuffed. One of my friends was a top solicitor and I even got him on the case, but there was nothing he could do, and the worst of it was that I was given no right of reply, so I didn't even get the chance to defend myself.

I was made to look like a conwoman.

It was a point in my life when I sat down and tried to figure out why it was that I seemed to keep ending up on the floor. Was I an easy target? Was I a sitting duck? What had I done to deserve this? All that I had tried to do was to better myself. I had made no great claims for Glyderm; the only mistake I had made was in allowing a woman to grind me down and to tell her something that I thought she wanted to hear. Why hadn't I gone with my gut instinct? Why hadn't I come right out and challenged her over her so-called acne?

I had worked so hard to get my life out of the gutter, and GM-TV had made me look like a con artist. I was devastated.

I moved out of 134 and briefly worked in an office at 10 Harley Street, but that didn't pan out, so I then decided to take the plunge and open my own salon, Hollywood Looks, in Harrow. It was 2000, and by this stage, Trevor, my brother, had established himself as an actor in Hollywood, and that is where the salon name came from. The salon was in a shopping centre and I was the first person to bring everything together under one roof – nails, cosmetic surgery consultations, skin peels, botox, fillers, the lot. We had three rooms, and the nail bar was fantastic. We also had a huge television on the wall – for once in my life,

I was ahead of the game and I seemed to have got something right.

We couldn't get customers through the door quickly enough. The place was heaving. But there was a downside, and that was the fact that I'd had to get Faisal involved because I couldn't quite afford to take it all on myself. So there was still that huge dark shadow in my life.

I believe that I might have become a millionaire through that business, but dear old Faisal was to have his say in that too...

CHAPTER 14
Made In Hollywood

I have alluded to my brother several times, and this is probably as good a juncture as any to tell you about him.

When Trevor and I were growing up, I always felt that my parents favoured him, although in later life the two of us would sit down and talk and he would say that he believed I was their favourite.

There was the usual sibling rivalry between us and we were never especially close, although he was always there for me if I needed him, and vice versa.

He announced one day that he was going to New York for a week's holiday. He went with a friend and at the end of the seven days the friend came back but Trevor decided to hire a car and drive to Los Angeles.

He fell in love with the place and decided to stay. Trevor was a professional boxer and he started picking up the odd fight in America and he was spotted by a talent scout, who told him that he thought he could get him some work in television adverts and suchlike.

True to his word, he got landed Trevor a Budweiser ad and he immediately realised that he could earn more for a few minutes work in front of a camera than he could for being in a boxing ring for 12 rounds. And, of course, he didn't have to stand there and take punches.

Trevor was bitten by the bug so he hired himself an agent to see if he could make a career out of acting in the United States. And the rest, as they say, is history. He hardly ever stopped working.

I went out to see him a few times with my daughters, Hannah and Charlotte, and we always had a great time when we were in LA. I also have to say that he was fantastic with the girls.

There was one trip where I had Faisal with me, and Trevor kept asking me why the pair of us didn't get married. "The pair of you really should get hitched, and why don't you do it in Vegas, while you are here?"

I kept telling Trevor that I didn't want to get married. I didn't want to go into all the reasons, and I certainly didn't want to explain to him about the way Faisal really was. Trevor really liked Faisal at first, but as the days went by he got to see more and more of what the man was like, and he couldn't help but hear that way that he spoke to me.

One of his worst quirks was at the dinner table. If Charlotte wouldn't eat all of her dinner, Faisal would tell her that not only wouldn't she get any dessert, but she wouldn't be allowed to eat again for ages. It was bizarre behaviour, and Trevor said so; all the more so because Faisal wasn't even her father.

On one occasion, Faisal went to the toilet, and while he was gone, Trevor ate Charlotte's dinner. He would wink at her and tell her not to say anything, and it became a standing joke between the three of us – every time we went out for a meal, Trevor would wait for Faisal to go to the toilet and then he would polish off Charlotte's dinner. I dread to think how much weight he must have piled on during that holiday. But that was the type of man my brother was.

Eventually, a combination of Trevor and Faisal wore me down and we ended up having a marriage ceremony in Las Vegas. I don't know why I allowed myself to be talked into it, but it wasn't the first thing I had done in my life that I later found difficult, if not impossible, to explain. We never registered our so-called 'marriage' in England, and I am certain that it wasn't a legal ceremony anyway.

Trevor got his first part in the TV series *Tour of Duty* in 1989, and after that the floodgates opened. Trevor appeared in a host of movies, including *Mortal Kombat, Men of War, Illegal in Blue, Deep Rising, Gone in 60 Seconds, Dead Man's Run* and, most famously, *Pirates of the Caribbean: The Curse of the Black Pearl*. He also appeared in a host of TV series, including *Murder, She Wrote, Baywatch, Nowhere Man* and *The X Files*, but his big break came when he landed the part of Lieutentant Commander Mic Brumby in *JAG* – between 1998 and 2001, he starred in 42 episodes. He also popped up in cult series such as *Friends* and *Frazier*.

Everybody assumed that I would be insanely jealous of Trevor's success. After all, I was the one who had wanted to be on stage, and I was the one who had tried and failed to be a performer. But I felt nothing but pride for him and everything that he achieved.

He met and married Ruth-Anne and they had two sons, Travis and Daniel, and he lived in Hollywood. Eventually he had an affair and Ruth-Anne filed for divorce.

Tragically, Trevor got involved in the drugs scene while he was in Hollywood and on 7 June, 2003, his girlfriend walked into the home they shared and found him dead on the floor. The autopsy declared that he didn't have enough drugs in his system to kill him, but there is little doubt in my mind that they caused his death. My parents chose not to believe it.

It was a horrific time, all the more so because Trevor had everything to live for. He was just 40 years old.

I was living in St Neots in Cambridgeshire at the time and the phone rang at 5am. I froze, because nobody calls you at that time unless it is with bad news. I'd had a premonition, and the second the phone started ringing, I knew that I was going to be told my brother had died. Sure

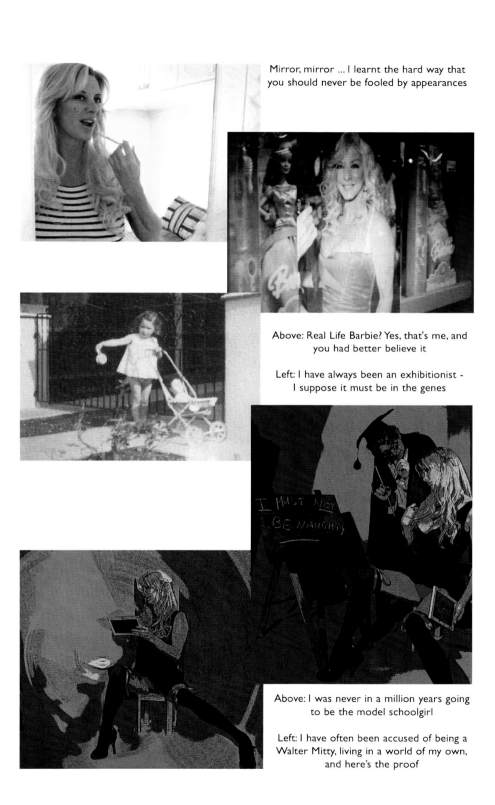

Mirror, mirror ... I learnt the hard way that you should never be fooled by appearances

Above: Real Life Barbie? Yes, that's me, and you had better believe it

Left: I have always been an exhibitionist - I suppose it must be in the genes

Above: I was never in a million years going to be the model schoolgirl

Left: I have often been accused of being a Walter Mitty, living in a world of my own, and here's the proof

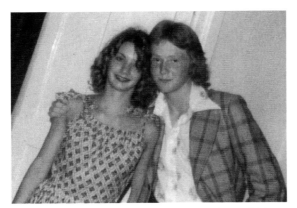

And to think, I used to be such a nice girl - aged 14, with Tony, the love of my life

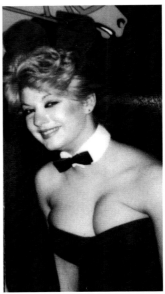

I was one of the original Playboy bunnies, and I loved every single minute of it

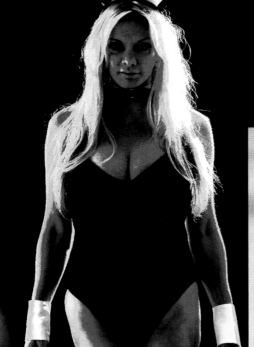

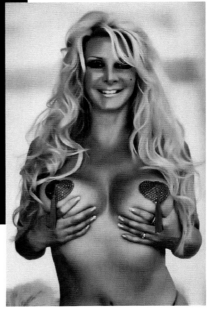

Above: "Sarah, you're fired!" I walk off into the sunset, thrown out on my bunny ears

Right: "Go on girl, show us your tits". It has been a common theme throughout my life and I figure that if you've got it, you may as well flaunt it

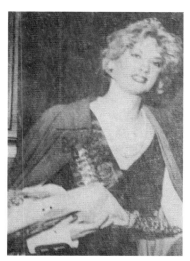

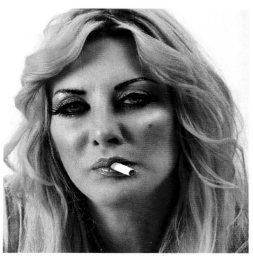

It could have been me. It should have been me - take that look off your face

Who loves ya baby? You may find this hard to believe, but I was a genuine gangster's moll

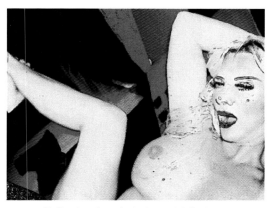

Coffee break with the boss didn't always go according to plan ...

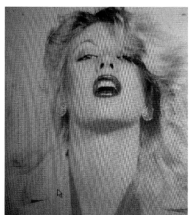

Marilyn Monroe eat your heart out - this town ain't big enough for the two of us

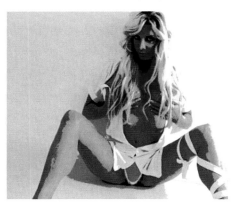

"This will look great in your portfolio Sarah. Of course everybody takes their clothes off for the photographer." A lucky escape from the casting couch

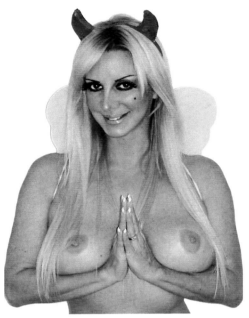

Butter wouldn't melt in my mouth. Don't you think I look like an angel?

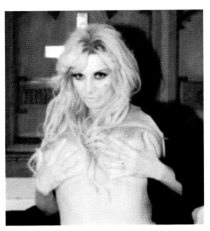

Doing God's work! Forgive me father for we are both about to sin

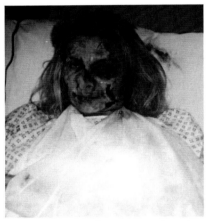

Battered beauty. Beaten to a pulp and dumped in the street by the man I loved

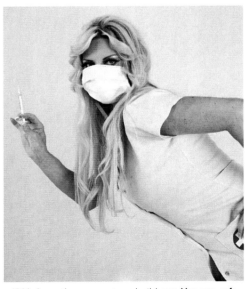

"We have the power to rebuild you. You are safe in our hands." In most respects, the NHS did a good job of patching me up

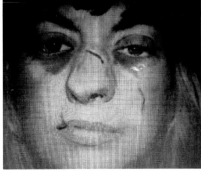

I wasn't exactly thrilled to bits with the way my nose looked after my beating

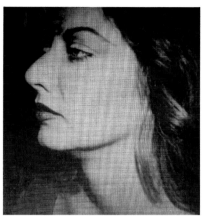

I was determined that things would improve - cosmetic surgery is a wonderful thing. But not when carried out by the NHS

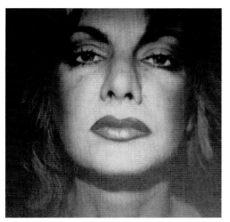

This was not what I had in mind when they told me that they would give me a nose job

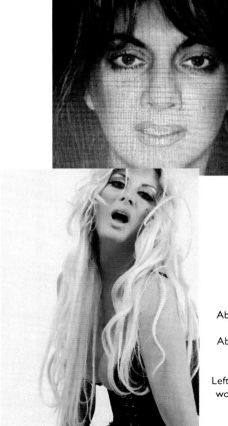

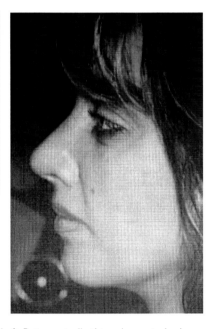

Above Left: But eventually things began to look up

Above Right: I was unhappy with the work carried out on me by the NHS - wouldn't you be?

Left: I am back! It took a long time, and a lot of hard work, but I was finally happy with the way I looked

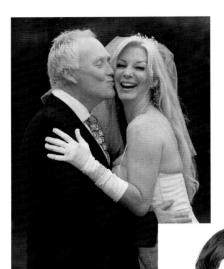

Happy ever after. Paradise is a feeling not a place, and I experienced it when I married Tony Burge

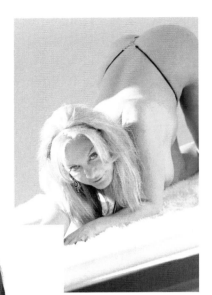

I was accused of being a benefits cheat in order to fund a new bum. What a cheek!

Meet the family. My beautiful daughter Charlotte, the designer, model and fashionista, and a girl who is going places

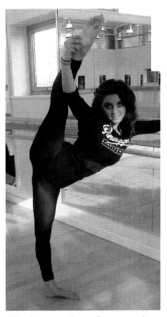

That's got to hurt. But not when you are a teenager. Daughter Hannah, who was born to dance

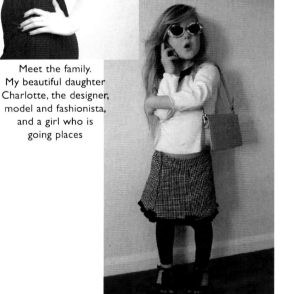

Last but by no means least - Poppy the diva, a gift of pure joy for Tony and I

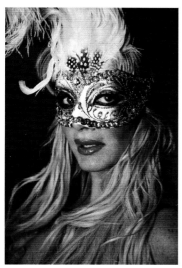

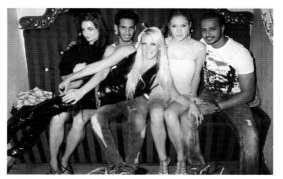

It's time to party. At one of my Madame Pink soirees with my daughter Charlotte, a prince from Abu Dhabi and some friends

The girl behind the mask - enter the one and only Madame Pink, a figment of a very naughty imagination

Mixing with the stars - with singer Alexander O'Neil at a Humanhi party

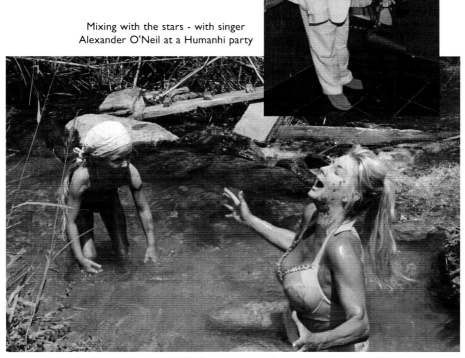

Splash it all over. Poppy and I filming on location for our own US reality TV show

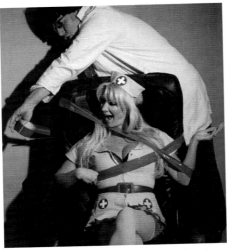

Carry on doctor. Having a bit of fun for the camera, making movies for the Japanese market

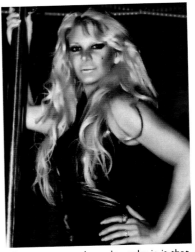

Driving me up the pole - why is it that some people have no sense of humour?

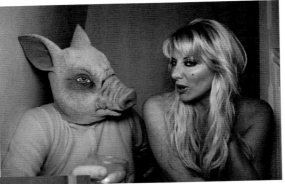

Pork scratchings! Don't even ask...

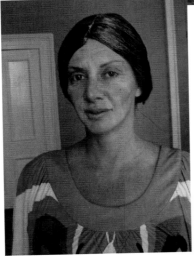

Beauty and the Beast, a reality TV show, gave me a glimpse of the way I never want to look

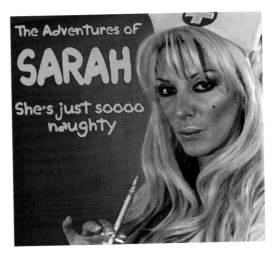

The Adventures of SARAH
She's just soooo naughty

enough, it was my Dad on the other end. All that he said was: "Trevor's dead."

I was numb. The feeling of emptiness inside is impossible to describe. I immediately recalled the bizarre telephone conversations I would have with him when he would phone me from America and announce that he was going to live forever. These were conversations that obviously took place when he was under the influence of whatever drugs he was taking.

On more than one occasion I told Trevor that if he wanted me to fly out to Hollywood to spend time with him, all that he had to do was ask, but he always said that things were fine. I later discovered that Dad went out to see him a couple of times, but nothing was ever said to me.

If the problem had been confronted head on then who knows? Trevor might still be alive. If I had known the full extent of the problem I would have been on the next flight out; even if it had meant getting him arrested, I would have done it if I had believed it would have helped to straighten him out.

His funeral was grotesque. There were cameras everywhere, and it felt like we were taking part in some sort of stage production. This was my brother's funeral, for Christ's sake.

It was held at the YMCA, where he went every day to train. It was a real spit-and-sawdust place. There were lots of actors present and I looked round at them and thought: "You are all fake. None of you give a damn about Trevor. You are just here to see if you can get yourself on the TV news tonight." No funeral is ever good, but this one was absolutely horrible.

I remember one of the members of the cast of *JAG* walking out to the front to deliver a tribute to my brother and asking: "Can everyone at the back hear me?" It was like he was putting on a performance. I looked around and it suddenly occurred to me that everybody was dolled up to the nines. It was a very ugly experience.

Dad got up to say his piece but he couldn't get the words out. It would have been bad enough anyway, but he was standing in front of a crowd of people he didn't know. I had been crying uncontrollably, but as I looked at this poor man I found an inner strength from somewhere and walked out to the front, took my Dad's hand and told him we would do it together. I spoke about the man I knew. It was at that point that I realised how truly awful my parents must have felt – it is not in the natural order of things for a parent to bury a child. My mother was so deeply affected by it that she couldn't face going.

That first service had been organised by Ruth-Anne, but we then had to attend another one, organised by his girlfriend. Only in Hollywood – this one was attended by most of the cast of *Pirates of the Caribbean* and was a totally different affair. It seemed to me that everybody had made up their minds they were going to get drunk and have sex, and that's pretty much what happened. Trevor would have approved.

Trevor Etienne, who was one of the pirates in the film, made a play for me and wanted to take me back to his hotel. Fortunately, my father stepped in and told me that I was going back with him – you do strange things where you are grieving, and Dad probably saved me from myself.

His ashes remain in an urn in a garage in Hollywood because his wife cannot bring herself to scatter them at sea, as he wished.

CHAPTER 15
The End Of A Nightmare

Meanwhile back in Harrow... Hollywood Looks, my one-stop beauty shop, was going great guns. I was especially proud of the fact that I had used my Harley Street contacts and been able to persuade some of the plastic surgeons to carry out consultations at the salon. They also performed some very minor procedures, such as applying botox. The whole concept was way ahead of its time.

From the day we first opened the doors the place was a huge success. Women could come in, perhaps feeling pretty low about their appearance, and we could give them some botox or a skin peel, sort out their nails, and they would walk out feeling like a million dollars. I swear to you that some of my customers used to grow a couple of inches, such was the effect of restoring a little self-confidence.

They would come into the salon with the weight of the world on their shoulders, and would leave the place floating on air. And in between, they had parted with a healthy amount of their husbands' hard-earned cash. Everyone was a winner!

When we were at our busiest, I employed 12 staff. It was all pink and purple and was very girlie.

The salon was five minutes away from my home in Pinner, which meant I could easily do the school run and still get to work before 9am. I loved it.

We stocked all the top products, I was my own boss and I was earning serious money. I knew that I had stumbled onto something special, so I also began to start thinking about setting up a chain of Hollywood Looks salons. The sky was the limit – London was plenty big enough to accommodate several more, and then there was the rest of the country.

Had I finally done something right? Could this really be happening to me? I was living my dream – and it was my dream. Nobody else could ever take any credit for this.

We bought non-surgical facelifting machines which, although they resembled instruments of torture, worked very well indeed, and we quickly built up a following of women who were eager to try them. And there were special machines that treated specific medical conditions, such as Bell's Palsy – this is a condition where the sufferer can lose control of facial muscles, and it is quite common for one side of the face to drop. But we had a machine that specifically designed to help those poor women.

From day one, I had been determined that this was something that I was going to do properly, so I hired a PR company and they took control of my advertising and publicity campaign, and we also invited the beauty editors from the leading magazines to come along, have a look and try out some of the treatments. We were absolutely switched on and I knew how to play the game to get the best possible return.

When we opened the place we had a proper launch party, which set the tone for everything that followed.

All was well in my world, but after about six months I would go to bed at night and dream about Tony Burge, my childhood sweetheart. Throughout my life I have had premonitions about various things, and I started to get this very strong feeling that Tony was out there somewhere, trying to find me.

The harder I fought it, and the more I tried to ignore it, the stronger the feelings became. I would go to work, come home and the moment I went to bed I would get this sensation again, that he was trying to find me.

I confided in my best friend, Karen Deacon, and she said: "Well what are you waiting for then? Just get in touch with him." I wanted to, I really wanted to, but I couldn't because years had passed since I last saw him, and I hadn't the first idea where he was living.

These feelings persisted for weeks, and eventually I was thinking about Tony all the time, when I was wide awake, when I was trying to go to sleep and again in my dreams when I finally nodded off.

Karen asked me what I was going to do. I have never done things by half, and briefly considered trying to locate him through Friends Reunited, but then I thought: "Blow that. I am going to hire a private detective." And that's what I did. I thumbed through *Yellow Pages*, found a likely candidate, handed over £300 up front and gave him all the details I could, such as his full name, his date of birth, the names of his parents and where he had grown up. What I didn't know at that point was that he was married, but that is another story.

And then I went home and waited. I don't know what I expected to happen next, but a couple of days later the private detective called me at work to tell me that he had found Tony.

"Now what do I do?"

"Well why do you want to see him?"

"That's none of your business. I paid you to do a job and you have done your job, so everybody should be happy."

"I understand that, but I need to make a note for my records."

"He's been trying to find me."

"How do you know that?"

"It doesn't matter how I know that, just give me his phone number or his address or whatever it is that you have."

"I've got his work number."

"Okay, let me have that please."

"Do you want to know anything else?"

"Anything else like what?"

"Like whether he is married."

It simply hadn't occurred to me that he would be married, but then again, why wouldn't he have met somebody and settled down? I mean, I had tried it often enough, and I still couldn't get it right.

But I told the detective that I wasn't interested in knowing anything like that. All I wanted was a number where I could get hold of him, speak to him and find out whether he really had been trying to locate me. I was given Tony's number at 3pm and waited until 5pm, as I was about to close the salon, and then I dialled his number.

My heart was almost jumping out of my chest. What was I going to say? What would he say?

The phone rang, and when it was answered, it was Tony's voice on the other end. I was thrown, and found myself asking for his address. "Who wants to know?" came the reply.

"It's Sarah."

"Not Sarah Goddard from Bromley?"

"Yes."

"My God, I've been trying to find you for months. I have been through Friends Reunited, and I have all the boys in my office trying to find you. I can't believe you have rung me."

As it turned out, Tony had done pretty well for himself, and was running his own aluminium supply business in a place called Dry Drayton in Cambridgeshire. But when he told me that he had been trying to track me down it made the hairs on the back of my neck stand on end. This was utterly surreal.

We had a long conversation, during which he told me that his Dad had died, and I was genuinely upset to hear that. He told me that his Mum was well, and suddenly we were chatting away like the old friends we were. It was as if we had never been apart. I told him about the salon, and we got talking about the respective cars that we both drove. Tony drove a Jaguar with a personalised number plate, and it was that plate that had allowed the private detective to find him so easily.

He then revealed that he was married and had two daughters, and I told him about my situation, and then he asked the fateful question.

"Sarah, are you happy?"

"It's a long, long story Tony, and not something I want to discuss over the phone. I will explain it all when I see you."

"And what makes you think that you are going to see me?"

He suggested that we meet up at a wine bar near Berkeley Square in London, but he wanted the meeting to happen ten days later. "Ten days? Why ten days?" As always, I didn't want to wait. I wanted to meet him right there and then.

I suggested that we hook up that evening but he said that he couldn't, that he would have to work out a way to get away from his wife because she was very possessive and wanted him to account for his every movement.

And so it was that we eventually did meet up ten days later. He told his wife one pack of lies, and I told Faisal another. I managed to persuade him that I was going to a beauty seminar, and he didn't suspect a single thing.

I cancelled all my appointments for the day and set off for my assignation. We had arranged to meet at midday but we were both early, and when I walked in he was standing at the bar. Although I had seen him a couple of times since we were teenagers, my image of Tony was still of this young boy, and I wasn't sure what he would look like now. But I couldn't wait to see him again.

Suddenly, I suffered a panic attack and dived into the ladies' toilets, hoping that he hadn't seen me, but he had. When I emerged, he got up, walked over to me and his first words were: "God, I have missed you so much Sarah. I have missed you all my life." With that, he puts his arms round me and gave me the biggest cuddle. It was so warm, and he was so caring, and at that instant I realised how much I had missed him too. It was a magical moment that neither of us would ever forget.

He later said: "When I caught sight of this vision out of the corner of my eye going straight into the toilets I knew that it just had to be you. I knew that you would want to check yourself out in the mirror first of all, just to make sure that everything was in place. And do you know what Sarah? It is. You look fantastic."

The two of us picked up where we had left off all those years before. It was as if all the rubbish that had happened to me had disappeared. We talked for hours, expressing regret that we hadn't remained together, and I told him about my two marriages, and then I told him about Faisal – everything about Faisal, and what he had done to me.

Tony was horrified. As I was telling him about the night of the attack, the tears rans down his cheeks. It was almost as if he felt guilty in some sort of mad way. "Why didn't you contact me? Why didn't you phone me, right then? You know that I would come and taken you away and that I would have looked after you and nursed you back to health.

"I would have had you sorted out. I am not short of money, Sarah, so I could have got you to the best plastic surgeons. Why, why, why didn't you get in touch with me?"

"It didn't enter my head to do so Tony. The way I figured it was that I had made my bed and I had to be prepared to lie in it. Besides, I had no idea you felt that way about me. Don't forget that you were the one who dumped me."

"But we were kids back then, and I didn't really know what I wanted. Besides, when you met up with me when you were married to Glenn, you must have realised then how I felt about you."

"I didn't. I honestly didn't. I just thought that was all about getting together for old time's sake. Besides, I didn't want you to see me like that."

And then it all came pouring out. "You have wasted all these years, and I have wasted all these years. I am with a woman I don't love, and you are with a man you don't love. Jesus Christ, I even had an affair with a woman just because her bloody name was Sarah. It was the closest that I could get to you. Then I had a child by somebody else. The money I have spent on divorce – if only I had known it at the time, you and I should have always been together. We were meant to be together. We have wasted far too many years. I have spent most of my adult life regretting not being with you. I have always missed you.

"There have been times in my life when all I have thought about has been you, Sarah."

And I had to admit that it had been the same for me. So maybe he was right. Maybe we were meant to be together. No matter what, I sure as hell couldn't explain those feelings I'd experienced before I tracked him down. How on earth could I possibly have known that he was trying to find me? There had to be some sort of connection between the pair of us.

With Tony I felt comfortable, at my ease. I didn't have to stop and think before I opened my mouth, didn't have to worry about saying the wrong thing. And he made me laugh. For too much of my adult life, I had forgotten what it was like to laugh. Everything always seemed so grim, so deadly serious, so frightening.

He told me that he had no intention of going back home to his wife that night, and I admitted that I felt the same way. But Faisal was expecting me home, so I had to phone him and tell him that I'd met a friend at the seminar, we'd had a few drinks and I was too drunk to come home. I told him I was going to stay with my friend. "You'd better come home," he said. But I'd made up my mind, and repeated that I really was too drunk. Grudgingly, he accepted it, but warned me that I had better not be back late the following morning.

So Tony and I booked a hotel room and made up for lost time. There was an interesting postscript to it all. It turned out that he had inadvertently dialled a number on his mobile phone and the person on the other end heard much of our conversation and the sex we had together. Thankfully, it wasn't his wife. It was one of his friends from work.

Obviously, we didn't realise somebody was listening in. When we got to the hotel, Tony asked me if I wanted a coffee, to go dancing or to have sex, and I said: "Oh, all three please."

"You haven't changed then."

Needless to say, we did not emerge from the hotel room. When he next went into the office, his mate said: "Hi Tony. Would you like a dance?"

"What are you talking about?"

"Or would you like coffee, or would you prefer sex?"

It freaked him out. "What the hell are you going on about?"

"You had a good time with her didn't you? With Sarah."

When he related the tale to me, I could imagine the colour draining from his cheeks. How could they possibly know?

Then his mate spilled the beans. "I've got it all on my phone Tony. Thank God it wasn't your wife who got the call, or else I have a funny feeling that you might have had your balls cut off by now."

So what happened next in my life?

I had to go home to my children. As far as everybody was concerned I'd been away for a day and a night, but it was all to do with business, and until I decided what I was going to do next, I had to keep up the pretence. The last thing on earth I needed was for Faisal to suspect that I was seeing another man.

It wasn't easy. Tony started phoning and texting me on a regular basis, and I would phone him whenever I could. Then there were the clandestine meetings. We snatched whatever time together that we could.

Tony made it clear that he wanted me out of the house in Pinner. "You have got to leave that man," he said. "I will look after you now. You wouldn't let me do it before, but I can do it now."

I wanted to go with him, but there were my children, Charlotte and Hannah, and there were belongings that I wanted to take with me. I knew that I couldn't tell Faisal I was leaving him because he had always told me that if I tried to leave him he would kill me. That meant everything had to be planned. If I was going to move out, it had to be when Faisal wasn't about.

"Maybe we should just see each other for a while and see how things develop. You might get sick of me, and decide that you don't want me after all."

"That is not going to happen Sarah. You have to trust me. I will not let you down and I will not let your daughters down."

The reality is that I was scared of what Faisal might do, especially if I took his daughter away from him without his prior knowledge. He had almost killed me once before, and on that occasion I hadn't done anything wrong. If I gave him just cause to lose his temper, there was no knowing how he might react.

I owed him nothing. Nothing at all. Apart from what he had done to me, there was also the time when he wanted to stand back and do nothing after Charlotte had been subjected to the most horrendous ordeal.

Faisal's father, Salah, had come over from Egypt after the death of his wife. He was in his late sixties and was a desperately sad man who was taking anti-depressants. I hardly knew this man – I had met him when we went on holiday to Egypt and stayed with him and his wife, although even that was a nightmare. I had been pregnant with Hannah at the time we visited them, and during our holiday I felt absolutely awful and suffered awful stomach pains – Faisal was as sympathetic as ever, accusing me of ruining our holiday.

Anyway, I welcomed Salah into my home because I felt sorry for him. He had nobody back home to share his life with.

At the time, Hannah was about two years old and Charlotte was 12. He took an immediate shine to Charlotte, and the two of them would play cards together, and she would show him pictures of London and tell him which places he should visit. She even offered to be his tour guide.

Although the two of them got on like a house on fire, I was wary of leaving them alone together. When all was said and done, this man was a stranger to both myself and my daughter.

One day I had to go and pick up Hannah from nursery school, and Faisal said that he wanted to come with me. I asked Charlotte if she also wanted to come along but she said no, she would stay at home with Faisal's father.

While we were collecting Hannah I began to feel uneasy. It is difficult to put my finger on it, but let's just say that I had a premonition that something wasn't right back at the house. I become highly agitated, and Faisal wanted to know what on earth was up with me.

"There's something wrong back at home, I know there is."

Naturally, he told me to relax and insisted that everything would be absolutely fine.

I was having none of it. We rushed back home and the second I walked into the lounge I knew that my instincts had been correct. Faisal's father was there, but there was no sign of Charlotte. I knew this man had done something unspeakable to my daughter. He was sitting there, all hot and sweaty, looking as guilty as sin.

I rushed upstairs to Charlotte's bedroom and she was lying there in floods of tears. I asked her what had happened and she told me that they had been sitting talking when he had put his arm around her shoulder and had started fondling her breasts. My daughter was 12 years old!

I didn't wait to hear anymore, but flew down the stairs, went into the kitchen and grabbed a knife and then I held him by the throat and totally lost the plot. "You bastard," I screamed. "You abused my daughter. I am going to fucking kill you."

Faisal, who had been in the kitchen, came into the lounge and pulled me off his father, demanding to know what I was doing.

"I am calling the police," I screamed. "Get this pervert out of my house. Get him out before I kill him."

"If we call the police, the only person who is going to be taken away is you Sarah. They are going to cart you off to the nut house. Get a grip. Who is going to believe you?"

I tried to calm down, to make some sense of all this ugliness, and tried to understand what had happened.

Faisal said: "If the police come, they will take Charlotte away from you because they will think you have neglected her. They will think it is unsafe for her to be here."

I realised that he might be right. "Okay, I will not call the police, but I want your father out of my house this instant."

"Sarah, we don't know the full story."

"I do know the full story."

By now I had his father pinned against the wall again and I told him to admit what he had done. He pretended not to understand what I was saying.

Then Faisal asked his father what he had done, and he finally admitted that he had interfered with Charlotte, although he said that it must have been the tablets he was taking that had made him do it. Jesus Christ – had this poor child of mine not been through enough in her short life?

Faisal's brother lived nearby, and ended up taking him in. Faisal made his brother promise not to tell his wife why I had kicked his father out of our home, but that only made me even angrier because they had two children of their own. I asked Faisal if he was totally insane, and took it upon myself to tell the wife what had happened. Needless to say, she wanted nothing to do with this man either.

"Well where's my father going to go?"

"I don't give a toss where he goes."

He ended up moving into a hotel, but still Faisal wouldn't let it go. "Wait until I tell your parents that you have thrown my father out of our home."

"Are you serious?"

In the end, I phoned my parents and told them I had thrown him out, and I explained why I had done so. They didn't want to know. It was another case of sweeping things under the carpet.

"Are you sure that's what happened Sarah?" said my Mum. "How do you know that's what happened?"

"I am sure it happened because Charlotte told me it happened, and she does not make up things like that. And I know it happened because he admitted doing it."

"I can't talk to you when you are like this Sarah. You are so dramatic."

"Mum, I want to come and stay with you for a while. I want to bring my children and I want to stay with you."

"Oh no, you've made your bed, so you have to lie in it."

And with that, she put the phone down.

I later discovered that he had tried to put his hands inside Charlotte's knickers and had only been distracted by a knock on the door which allowed her to break free and run upstairs to her room. I dread to think what could have happened.

Eventually I took Charlotte to the doctor because I just wanted somebody to listen to me. And he more or less confirmed what Faisal had said, namely that Charlotte might well have been taken into care until the matter had been resolved. That would probably have been the final straw, so thank God the police were not dragged into it.

Faisal's father was finally put on a plane and sent back to Egypt, and I tried my best to erase all memories of him from my brain. Then, a few years later, Faisal said: "Right then, Dad's landing from Egypt in a few hours and I am going to pick him up from the airport and bring him back here. Will you try to be nice to him please?"

"Nice? You are asking me to be nice? You expect me to welcome this man back into my home after what he did to Charlotte?"

"Well he's coming, and that's an end to it."

"Let me try to explain this to you in a way that you will understand – if that man sets foot in my home, I will stab him. And that is a promise."

"Then you will go to prison."

"I am begging you not to do this."

But he did do it, so I took my children and we cleared off to Alton Towers, with me telling Faisal that I wouldn't be back until his father was gone. Faisal got the message, and within a few days his father had moved out and went to stay with his other son, even though his wife knew what had happened all those years previously. By now, it wasn't my problem.

So, why would I have any second thoughts about leaving this man?

No matter what Tony said, no matter how often he assured me that he would be able to protect me from this man, I couldn't quite come to terms with the thought of walking out. Yes, I had tried to build up an escape fund, but that was when I was going to leave him and go and live on my own with the girls. This would be very different. I would be leaving him to go and live with another man.

Faisal was the most jealous and possessive individual I had ever met. If he thought I had been sleeping with another man behind his back, there was no imagining what he might be capable of doing. And I wasn't just scared for myself. I was frightened for my daughters, and I was afraid of what he might do, or have done, to Tony. I could live with many things on my conscience, but if anything had ever happened to Tony because of his relationship with me, I don't know what I would have done.

Tony wasn't scared of Faisal, and he was quite prepared to face the consequences, whatever they might be. I remember sitting in his car one day, not far from where I lived, and he said: "Come with me now, right now. Forget about your clothes – I can afford to buy you a new wardrobe, and I can afford to buy new clothes for the girls. Come with me now, and we will pick up the girls from school and we will be gone before anybody knows what has happened."

Don't forget that I had also built up a successful business. If I went with Tony, I realised that I would have to leave Hollywood Looks. It had taken me many years to get on my feet, and here I was at a point where I was financially independent, bringing in good money, having come up with this great idea. Could I bring myself to walk away from it all for the man whom I now knew truly was the love of my life, the man I was supposed to be with?

"Do I stay with Faisal, coin it in from the business and have an affair on the side, or do I follow my heart and settle down with Tony?"

He had no such doubts. Tony decided that he couldn't cope with having a secret affair, so he went home one day and told his wife that he was leaving her because he had been reunited with his childhood sweetheart. She was dumbfounded. It must have felt she had been felled by an axe, all the more so because she didn't see it coming. He told her that he had never really loved her, and that must have hurt like hell.

He was on a roll now, and also admitted that, while they had been married, he'd had an affair, and as a result of that he had fathered a child. Talk about a bolt from the blue.

With that, he turned on his heels and walked out. He then phoned me and said: "Hello Sarah, I have done something that I think you ought to know about. I have told Rebecca everything, and I do mean everything. So I have now moved out and am going to stay with my mother for a while, but the ball is now in your court. Are you coming with me?"

On one hand, I was thrilled that he cared so much about me that he had sacrificed everything in order to get me; on the other, my stomach was churning. Now I would have to make the decision. Fobbing him off was not going to be an option. Tony had made it quite clear that he was not going to be fobbed off, that he expected me to leave Faisal, leave the salon and begin a new life with him.

I knew that Tony would not let it rest, and there was also the thought that Rebecca would either get hold of my phone number or find out where I lived, and come round and kick up a stink. And who could have blamed her? As far as she was concerned, I had destroyed her marriage; never mind the fact that long before I had reappeared on the scene he had seen fit to have an affair that produced a child.

Finally I made my decision. We were going to go. I phoned up the mother of Hannah's best friend and asked if she could possibly look after Hannah for me for a day or so. I briefly explained that I was planning to leave Faisal and that I was terrified of how he would react and didn't want my daughter to be exposed to it, so the mother agreed. Charlotte was about 17 years old by this point, and she was delighted that I'd finally found somebody who loved me. She was happy to move into a flat with a friend.

I wasn't thinking about packing huge numbers of suitcases or anything like that, and there was no question of calling in a removal man to take my treasured bits and pieces of furniture.

You would, I am certain, understand if I had decided to do all this behind his back, but that wasn't my style. I wanted this man to know what was happening. I did not want him to come home to an empty house and wonder where I was. In saying that, I waited until he was in the kitchen, making himself some toast or whatever, and went to the front door. Just before I slammed it shut I shouted: "I just want you to know that I am leaving you."

With that, I ran to Tony's waiting car, leaving with the clothes I stood up in and very little else. Within seconds my mobile phone was ringing. It was him.

"What do mean you are leaving me? Where are you? What are you doing? Are you mental?"

"No, anything but. I have left you, and I will not be coming back. I have met somebody else, somebody who treats me properly, with respect. You have made my life a misery. You are nothing but a fucking bully, and I hate you with all my heart. I can't describe how much I hate you. I had to pretend to love you for years, just so that I could pacify you, but now it's over. I'm gone."

"You are insane. Are you insane? You get back here right now because we are going to sort this out."

"Don't you understand what I am telling you? I hate you, and I have done for years. I have left you. I am not coming back."

After that, the shit really hit the fan. Rebecca managed to get hold of my home phone number, so she ended up getting hold of Faisal, and you can imagine the conversations they had about Tony and I. They managed to convince themselves that they were the true victims in all of this. I can tell you for certain that Rebecca was never thrown down a flight of stairs. She was never kicked and punched; she didn't end up with a broken jaw, broken eye sockets, a punctured lung and a smashed nose. She wasn't raped by the man who supposedly loved her. So you will forgive me, I am sure, if I admit that I found it hard to summon up much sympathy for Rebecca.

Then we found out that Faisal was on the phone to Rebecca's mother. How on earth that came about, or what he hoped to achieve from it, I will never know. It was bonkers.

While all of this was going on, Tony and I had to decide where we were going to live. He had a boat at Port Solent in Portsmouth. Our mobile phones hardly stopped ringing, and my parents disowned me for about the one-millionth time. My father would at least talk to me, but Mum refused. There she was again, brushing things under the carpet.

I explained to Dad that Faisal had been a bully and a thug throughout our relationship. He hit me, he beat me up, he spat at me – why the hell would they want me to stay with a man who was capable of inflicting that sort of torture upon their only daughter? Why were they siding with him, not with me? They were consoling Faisal, the victim. And there he was, telling them that I was the one who had been hitting him. It seemed that they took his word over mine. How could that be?

There was a telephone conversation with my father in which he said: "Sarah, how could you? What you have done to that man is wrong." I couldn't understand why nobody was listening to me. Not even my own parents. This was a man who on one occasion pulled a revolving window into my face and knocked me out cold. This was a man who had broken just about every bone in my body at various times. And this was a man who had told me that he would kill me.

It was awful. But through it all, I had Tony, and I was convinced that I had made the right choice, that for once my decision had not been flawed. I also tried to convince myself that my family would come around. There was one small consolation in all of this, and that was the support that we got from Tony's mother.

She told him: "You have done the right thing. Rebecca was never right for you anyway, so it is best that you are out of that relationship. If you are in love with Sarah, and you obviously are, then you should give yourselves the opportunity to make this work. These chances don't come along too often."

So at least we had the blessing of one person who mattered to us both.

In all of this, there was the salon. I knew that I couldn't just leave it. Apart from anything else, I had responsibilities to the people who worked there. Naturally, by the time I got to the salon, Faisal had given everybody his version of events. He was the one who had been wronged, and I was the evil witch.

I couldn't work in an atmosphere like that, and I certainly couldn't work in a salon where Faisal would frequently come in unannounced and do everything within his power to belittle me. Tony was brilliant throughout all of this, and said that he would buy out Faisal because he knew how passionate I was about the business.

We consulted lawyers and accountants and put a figure on the business and Tony then went to see Faisal to see whether they could work out a deal, but he didn't want to know. I think that if we had offered him £20m he would still have turned us down flat because he didn't want to see me happy.

"Over my dead body will she get anything out of this business," he said. "I will burn it to the ground first." And he would have done.

One of Tony's friends had a lorry and in the end, we turned up one day and decided to start dismantling the salon, salvaging whatever we could. I was determined that I was going to walk away with something, but this would never have been the route that I would have chosen, and I was in floods of tears as I watched my dream being taken apart and thrown in the back of a lorry.

At least I walked away with the tools of my trade.

While all of this was going on, Tony's Jaguar was badly vandalised, and I started receiving death threats on my mobile from men with Eastern accents who announced that they were going to kill me. I was scared. Really scared. The pressure on us was unrelenting.

Tony eventually rented a house in Welwyn Garden City and I moved in there with the girls, hoping that we could make a fresh start. But still the abusive phone calls and the threatening texts continued.

After a while I realised that there some personal possessions back at the house in Pinner that I wanted, so I went to collect them. I could have gone behind Faisal's back but I didn't, so I got in touch with him and arranged to meet him at the property.

As you can imagine, this was not an encounter that I was looking forward to. I was filled with trepidation, but I also knew that I couldn't back down, that I had to face him. Perhaps this would be the meeting that would bring everything to a conclusion, and we could all find a way to move forward.

Faisal promised that he wasn't going to hurt me, so I managed to persuade Tony to let me go on my own. He let me in and I went upstairs to get my clothes, but as I started to pick them up I realised that he had cut them up. They were all destroyed. I could have coped with that – they were just clothes, all of which could be replaced.

But what I found really difficult was realising that he had also destroyed all my children's toys and possessions. And the thing that finished me off was discovering that every personal photograph, every video, had either being ripped apart or smashed. It was as if my entire past had been wiped out. Apart from my memories, I had nothing left of my past life. There were no photographs of my brother, or of my daughters. Of all the things he had done to me, and there was plenty to choose from, this was perhaps the cruellest thing of all.

I was stunned. And the finishing touch was that the man who had done all of this, then fell to his knees and, crying like a baby, begged me to come back to him.

"I have loved you all this time," he said.

"No man who loves somebody treats them the way you have treated me."

"I promise I will change. I will become a better person, if only you will come back to me."

He probably meant it, but men like him never change.

"It's too late, far too late."

I knew that I needed to get out, but he was clinging on to me, begging me to stay. I have always been taught that, deep down, bullies are cowards, and his behaviour that day proved it to me beyond any doubt.

After I had left and got back to Welwyn Garden City, the old aggression and the threats returned with a vengeance. He called me every name under the sun, and a good many others too.

My business had gone and I had left my home, but at least I was with the person I loved, which was more important to me than anything else.

The thing that nagged away at me, however, was the fact that I had taken his daughter away from him. I was sure that he would want to see her, and my parents even contacted him to ask whether he wanted to see her. His response to them was: "Who is Hannah?" And he put the phone down. Now they knew what kind of man he was.

Funnily enough, that was the point when something seemed to click with him, and all the phone calls and the threats stopped. So I was rid of him at last.

This was a period in my life where I sat down and took stock, and where I considered everything he had put me through. It helped me to realise that I had definitely done the right thing.

I recalled some of the worst things he put me through. Like the time we were out for a meal and he accused me of looking at a man. I told him not to be stupid. When we went out for a meal – and this was meant to be a 'romantic' meal – I always preferred to sit across the table from the person I was with, but he always insisted on sitting next to me, and I hated it.

There were not many people in this particular restaurant, and the next thing I knew was that he had hit me in the face with his hand. And all because I was meant to be looking at somebody – if I had been sitting across the table from Faisal, then of course I would have been looking at him. I was stunned by what he had done, but the bastard was cute enough to make sure that nobody saw him do it.

Then there was the time that I had to go to hospital because I thought he had broken my ankle after jumping on it. It wasn't broken, but they put a plaster on it to give me some support. When I went home to him he said that he was sorry and that it would never happen again. He was always sorry, and he would always say that it would never happen again. Until the next time.

The time he struck me with the revolving window, he was inside the house and I was in the garden. He said something and we ended up arguing and I walked towards the window. As soon as I got within range, he spun the window with all his force and it struck me on the head and knocked me out cold. There was blood everywhere. I had to go to hospital and ended up with stitches above my eye where the window caught me – a fraction lower and I would have lost an eye.

I wasn't allowed to have friends, and I wasn't allowed to have nights out with the few friends that I did have. The only time that I could go out was when I could make arrangements that coincided with the nights where he was working and I wasn't. Charlotte would babysit Hannah for me, but I would have to swear her to secrecy, and make her promise that she wouldn't say a word to Faisal.

Sometimes I did some pretty stupid things. I dabbled in cocaine for the first and only time in my life because I wanted to know if it would dull the pain, and I had sex with other men, but the thing that gave me the biggest kick was that he didn't know. I felt that I was getting one up on him. And before Tony came back into my life, subconsciously I was probably hoping to meet the right man, somebody who would treat me properly.

Bizarrely, Faisal would time me when I did certain things. I would go off and do the shopping and when I would come back he would tell me that I had been away for, say, an hour and ten minutes.

"Why did it take you an hour and ten minutes?"

"What? I have been shopping, and that's the time it took, that's all."

"Why are you late? What have you been buying that took you so long?"

If ever I bought anything for Charlotte he would go nuts and ask me where I thought the money was coming from. He was insanely jealous of her because she a reminder of a love I'd had for somebody else. So whenever I got anything for her I would always have to tell her to hide it away.

It was the same with any clothes that I bought for myself. He would demand to know where they had come from, how much they had cost. In the end I would pretend that it was something I'd had for months, or I would tell him Mum and Dad had bought it for me, or that my friend Karen had bought it for me because she thought I would like it.

In a drunken stupor, he would often drag me into the outside garage at the back of our house and lock me in. He used to particularly relish doing this to me when the weather was freezing cold. I was treated worse than a dog by him.

Thank God for Tony.

My daughter has never seen her father since the day we walked out; nor does she want to.

Some years later, Veronica, his other daughter told Charlotte that Faisal had said that he might like to contact Hannah. She has turned 16, so the decision would be hers, and when I heard that he might want to get in touch I told Hannah.

"Oh yes Mum, so what am I going to say when he phones me. 'Hi Dad, how are you? And where, precisely, have you been all my life?' I don't think so. I have no desire to meet him or to talk him. Why would I want to?"

It is sad that a daughter should feel that way about her father, don't you think? But let's get one thing clear – this is a view she has formed all by herself, one that had nothing whatsoever to do with me. I have given her a telephone number where she could contact him if she so wished, and she also has Veronica's number, so the choice is hers and hers alone.

Faisal eventually remarried, to a woman much younger than himself. Her name is Sarah (really). And they have a son together.

I didn't have any contact with him for years but phoned him at work in 2010 because I wanted to ask him one final time if he really had destroyed all my photographs. He answered the phone and I said: "Hello Faisal, it's Sarah." He told me that I had the wrong number. It was bizarre. Anyway, I told him not to be so bloody stupid. There had been no contact between us for a very long time – if I had been in his shoes, my first thought would have been that something had happened to my daughter, but he didn't once mention her, not even to ask how she was.

"Faisal, this is important to me. Did you really burn and destroy all my photographs and videos? I have nothing to remind me of my brother, and neither do my parents. So did you destroy it all?"

"Go down to Harrow dump."

And those were the final words we ever exchanged.

CHAPTER 16
My Knight In Shining Armour

With my salon gone, I had no form of income and was entirely dependent upon Tony. It wasn't easy for him because he was supporting Rebecca, his lover's daughter, and me and my girls. That was pretty tough, even for somebody earning the sort of money he was at the time.

His company was called Railex Aluminium, and it was extremely successful. He told Rebecca that he wanted a divorce but she made it perfectly clear that she had no intention of making life easy for him.

We bought a five-bedroom house in St Neots. It was on an estate, which was something I had never experienced before, but I loved it. Tony had worked as a chef at the Savoy Hotel many years ago, so he was happy to do all the cooking, and I was madly in love with him.

By now we had put the wasted years behind us and were looking forward to the future and to making up for lost time. Because Railex Aluminium was his own company, Tony only went in to work when he felt that he had to, and he could do a lot of his business over the phone, so we spent a huge amount of time together in our little love nest. I was as happy as I had been at any stage in my life.

Yes, I was still simmering with some resentment that Hollywood Looks had been taken away from me, but it was only a beauty salon when all was said and done. Tony and I, that was real life.

Charlotte was 17 and she became a bit rebellious. Mind you, after everything that she had been through, my daughter was perfectly entitled to kick up her heels. Part of the problem may well have been that when I was with Faisal I used to try and shower her with attention because I didn't want to spend time with him – we would never, for instance, lie on the sofa and hold hands or have a kiss and cuddle. So all my affection went to Charlotte, and when I moved in with Tony she may have been a little bit jealous because I did want to lie on the sofa with him and hold hands and kiss and cuddle. It was very difficult for me to get the balance right, I can see that now.

Charlotte obviously felt left out. She was also totally bemused by the experience of seeing her mother walking around with a smile on her face. I tried to explain to her that I wasn't shutting her out, that all of this was new to me too.

She announced that she wanted to go to university, and ended up going to Nottingham to study fashion and design.

Hannah, meanwhile, was growing up into an intelligent, well-rounded young girl who worked hard at school, and who never spoke about her father. I sat her down and asked her if she felt that she needed to talk about him, but she assured me that she didn't. She soon established a circle of friends, nice people who never caused any problems.

We ended up with an extended family because Tony's daughters from his previous marriage used to come to stay with us, and then we were all introduced to the daughter he had conceived when he was having his affair. It was pretty complicated, but somehow we all managed to muddle along together. I don't want to paint this like it was some kind of fairytale because it most certainly wasn't that – there were rivalries between all these children and it was only natural that they would come to the surface from time to time. But we were able to cope, we were able to address the problems as they came along and we were usually able to solve them.

At last, there was no domestic violence in my life.

I had never known what it was like to live a normal life, and I realised that I enjoyed it. At one stage I even considered learning how to cook, but I quickly dismissed that idea. Well you know what they say about old dogs and new tricks. And, honestly, Tony never once complained about the fact that he had to do all the cooking.

The financial strain did take its toll in the end. As well as Tony was doing, there was a limit and we were fast approaching it.

I tried to hook up with a cosmetic surgery clinic in Huntingdon, outlining my qualifications, telling them that I used to work in Harley Street and that I'd had extensive plastic surgery myself. I knew how it worked, and I could talk to potential patients and put them at their ease and explain what each technique would involve.

They suggested that I might be able to help their marketing and publicity department and promised that somebody would get in touch with me to discuss how this might work.

In the meantime, I made up my mind that I was going to start working from home because I had all the tools of my trade that we had salvaged from the salon. I set up a room in the house and was in the process of researching advertising costs and working out which was the best local newspaper in which to advertise. I then had to source supplies all over again. It was a comedown – I had worked in Harley Street, and I'd had my own salon. But I was determined to make it work, and if there was only myself then maybe I could actually make a decent amount of money from it.

Personally, I was happy, Professionally, I wasn't.

Rebecca, Tony's wife, seemed to have made it her mission to clean him out, to relieve him of every penny he possessed. Money was tight, so while I was waiting for my business to get off the ground, I decided to claim benefits.

I explained my position, telling them that I was in the process of establishing a business, but they told me that wasn't a problem. I was given various forms to fill in and was informed that I would soon be receiving some money. It wasn't a fortune and it hardly scraped the surface, but I suppose that £67 a week was better than a slap in the face with a wet kipper.

Then I was informed that I was also entitled to housing benefit. As far as I was concerned, this was all legal and above board. I hid nothing from them and was 100% honest about everything. I was given another form to fill in and before I knew where I was, I was receiving housing benefit. In total, I was getting about £90 a week.

Unbeknown to me, I had been given an incorrect form to fill in, and that would come back to haunt me.

In the meantime, the cosmetic surgery hospital got back to me and asked me to come in and help them with their PR campaign. A double-page spread appeared in one of the Sunday newspapers, for which I received not one penny. The heading read something like: 'All I want for Christmas is a new bum'. The idea was that I was pretending to be a potential patient and the theme of the story was that I wanted my bum done, and I was going to have it done at the hospital in Huntingdon.

It was a publicity stunt. No more, no less. As far as I was concerned, it was going to help the hospital and maybe I might end up getting some work out of it. As it turned out, the article made next to no mention of the hospital but focused instead on the amount of cosmetic surgery I'd had – at the time, it amounted to somewhere in the region of £80,000.

I was described as a plastic surgery addict, which also implied that I had lots of money.

As my rotten luck would have it, somebody from the local social security office read the article and recognised me as the woman who had been in to claim benefits. "Hang on a minute, this woman has spent £80,000 on cosmetic surgery, and we are paying her housing benefits? That can't be right."

I may well have spent £80,000 on plastic surgery, but what that had to do with my life at this particular moment in time, I have no idea. For all they knew, I might have spent that money ten years before – what did it have to do with them anyway? It was none of their business, and it wasn't as if I had thousands of pounds hidden away.

The next thing I knew was that I had to appear before the social security's benefit fraud investigators, who accused me of claiming money illegally. I informed them that I had gone to the offices, asked for advice and had been given some forms to sign. End of story as far as I was concerned.

"But you spent £80,000 on plastic surgery."

"It is an article in a newspaper, and you really shouldn't believe everything that you read."

"How much did you get paid for the article? You didn't notify us that you received any payment."

"That's because I didn't get paid a penny. I was doing somebody a favour."

"Well we have it on good authority that you were paid £100,000."

"£100,000? What cloud are you on? That is utter nonsense. I have already told you that I was paid nothing, and that is the truth."

My benefit was suspended immediately, and then began an investigation that burrowed into my past and seemed to take for ever to resolve.

Initially, I wasn't too bothered because my business from home was taking off. On a smaller scale, I was offering the same sort of service that had been tied in with Hollywood Looks, so skin peels and that sort of thing. For local women it meant that they didn't have to travel to London to get this treatment; once again, I was the only person providing these services in this way.

Word of mouth quickly spread and before I knew what was happening, I was making a fortune, and the best part of it all was that because I was doing it from home, there were no overheads to worry about. It was perfect.

I was able to make my own hours, and ended up preferring it to the salon. At its peak, I was pulling in about £10,000 a week, but all the while I was still being investigated by the DSS and I was finally taken to court in 2005, where I was charged with benefit fraud. I couldn't quite believe that this was happening to me because as far I was concerned then – and now – I had done absolutely nothing wrong. Remember that the forms had been stuck under my nose, I had been told to sign them and I had signed them. If I was guilty of anything it was that I maybe should have checked those forms more thoroughly, but it never entered my mind for a second that I should have to and never in my worst nightmares did I think it would come to this.

Many things have happened to me throughout my life, but being branded a cheat and a liar was right up there with the worst. I am not totally stupid – people believe what they are told, and it is true that mud sticks, no matter what the circumstances. I was filled with horror at the thought that people I knew might think I had gone out of my way to defraud the benefit system. I was appalled at the thought that I would walk down the street and people would point at me and identify me as a benefits cheat. It was dreadful.

All this completely overshadowed one of the absolute highlights of my life. When Tony and I got together, our priority was to try to have a baby together – it was all the more important to us as a couple because of the abortion I'd had all those years before. We just felt that a child would make our relationship and our happiness complete, but I also knew that as I was approaching my mid-forties, it might not happen.

To complicate matters further, Tony had had a vasectomy, so the first thing we had to do was to get that reversed, and that wasn't straightforward either. The specialist we first saw looked more like the hospital cleaner than a highly-skilled surgeon, and I found it very hard to take him seriously, especially when he asked Tony to drop his trousers and then started flicking his penis with a pencil. It was one of the more bizarre sights that I had ever witnessed, so much so that I ended up getting a fit of the giggles, and Tony had to tell me to shut up and get a grip of myself.

We ended up calling the specialist "Dr Bollocks", but he certainly knew what he was doing and described in great detail what could be done to get Tony firing on all cylinders again. There were no 100% guarantees, but he was fairly confident, so we agreed to go ahead.

"Will it work?" Tony asked him.

"It should do."

"Well I tell what I will do – if it works, I will pay you, and if it doesn't, I won't."

"I will send you my bill Mr Burge and we will see what happens."

He had the operation and went straight back to work, even though he was walking like somebody who'd had a broom handle stuck up his backside. I wanted to start trying for a baby straight away, even though his bollocks were the size of footballs. He had been advised to wait at least three weeks for everything to heal properly before having sex. Bollocks to that! We were at it almost from day one, trying to make up for lost time.

We thought that, taking everything into account, it was a recipe for disaster and we would have no chance whatsoever of producing a baby between us. But I guess that it was just meant to be. After everything that Tony and I had been through, as individuals and as a couple, I discovered that I was pregnant and on 23 March, 2004, I gave birth to Poppy Honey, our wonderful daughter, and a special gift.

Meanwhile, I was accused of fraudulently claiming £1,700. It was hardly the crime of the century, even had I plotted to do it deliberately. The collapse of Barings Bank it was not.

I had to appear at Huntingdon Magistrates' Court. When I arrived, there were photographers everywhere. I was stunned by all this attention, but then I realised that the story was going to be written as me being a woman who was so heavily addicted to plastic surgery that I was prepared to defraud the benefits system to feed my habit. It was rubbish.

The bottom line was that because I had signed the wrong forms, through no fault of my own, I had no option but to plead guilty. I was livid. I tried to explain that it was an innocent mistake but nobody seemed to want to know anything about that.

The case was adjourned while they performed a series of background checks and suchlike to establish what they saw as a fit and proper punishment. I wanted the thing over and done with, but no, I would have to return for sentencing.

And guess when I had to make my second appearance in court? On 23 March, 2005. Poppy's first birthday. "Happy birthday darling. I am sorry about this, but Mummy has to go to court." Can you imagine it?

I asked my Mum to come and look after Poppy and I don't mind telling you that I was really scared. Previously, I had been quite confident that it would all be sorted out and that I might be given a slap on the wrists and a small fine, but because there had been such a media circus at the first hearing, I was convinced that the magistrates would want to make an example of me, so I returned to court filled with trepidation.

And this time there were even more photographers and journalists. It was bad enough that there were local media in court, but the tabloids had also sent people along, so the circumstances were perfect for them to hang me out to dry. I was later branded as the 'woman who cheated the benefits system to have a bum like Kylie'.

And apart from the printed media, local TV and radio were there in numbers too.

I was being prosecuted by a woman called Victoria Stevens, who recommended a custodial sentence to the magistrates. For £1,700! Was she having a laugh? I guess that she was loving her 15 minutes of fame.

"A custodial sentence is the only thing that will bring this woman to her senses," she said, and the whole thing turned into a debate about the rights and wrongs of plastic surgery. It was as if I was starring once more in my own personal horror movie.

I was given a chance to speak and I made it perfectly clear that I'd never had buttock implants, that no plastic surgeon had been anywhere close to my bottom. Would nobody believe me when I told them that it was just a media stunt, that I hadn't been paid for the story and that I really had been trying to do the clinic in Huntingdon a favour that backfired so spectacularly in my face?

Prior to 23 March, I had been required to speak to a probation officer, whose job it was to assess my character and, I guess, to work out what would be a fit and proper sentence for me, and I broke down during one of those sessions because I still couldn't understand why I was being prosecuted. Why would nobody listen when I told them that somebody at DSS had made the mistake, not me?

I admitted that I'd had plastic surgery, but tried to get them to accept that I'd had it years before, and that it had nothing to do with my claim. I tried to explain that I'd only wanted to claim the money to which I was entitled, and only until I got my business off the ground. And I tried to explain my personal circumstances, that I was living with a wonderful man, but that the demands on his finances had finally taken their toll. Nobody cared. Nobody wanted to listen.

"I haven't tried to defraud the benefit system, and if I had then I can assure you that I would have done it for rather more than £1,700," I said. "That would only buy you a few shots of botox, not bum implants."

Even the person who was assessing me admitted that she was stunned the case had gone to court.

But it had gone to court. At one point I looked around the Magistrates' Court and couldn't quite believe the numbers of people packed in. "My God," I thought. "This plastic surgery debate really does get people worked up."

Fortunately, the magistrates decided that they did not want to make an example of me. I can only believe that they saw through all the rubbish and believed that I had made a genuine mistake because they gave me a suspended sentence and ordered me to repay the £1,700. I thanked them, all the while thinking what a huge waste of time and money this had been.

My solicitor told me to leave court by the back entrance in order to avoid the waiting media scrum. The second Tony and I stepped out the door there was a camera in my face and I was being asked how it felt to cheat the benefits system. I put my hands up to my face and then the two of us ran off down the street with photographers, cameramen and journalists in tow. It was like a scene from *Bonnie and Clyde*.

Eventually Tony snapped and told them to leave us alone. We managed to put some space between them and us, and they gave up the chase, so we dived into a local pub and there was a TV switched on – and it was showing Tony and I running down the road.

My home phone didn't stop ringing for days, and we had journalists camped outside the house, all wanting their exclusive. We had magazines and newspapers queueing up wanting to talk to me. But they didn't want to talk to me about the court case – they were only interested in the plastic surgery.

I spent days in tears. Obviously, my business had been flushed down the pan again. I had worked so hard to establish it, and suddenly it was all gone. You may wonder why, but who were people going to believe? Were they going to believe the newspapers that branded me a benefits cheat or were they going to believe me when I told them I had inadvertently signed the wrong form when it was put in front of me? I will give you a clue – they were going to believe the newspapers.

I had been doing so well from my little room at home, but they even took that away from me, and so I had to try and dust myself down and find a way of starting all over again. How many times?

Throughout my life, every time I have built up or established something worthwhile, somebody has come along and taken it away from me. I know that I can be a little naïve sometimes, and that I am often too trusting of people, but I never seem to learn. And that simply makes every disappointment in my life hurt that little bit more. Each time it happens, a little piece of you is destroyed.

To make matters worse, as if they could ever get any worse, Tony's ex-wife was back trying to get more money from him. Everywhere we turned, an accusing finger was being pointed, and I admit that I wallowed in my misery for a while, and shed a great many tears and spat a lot of feathers, but then I woke up one morning and I thought: "I will be damned if I am going to let you lot batter me any more. I have had enough of this. I am going to make the most of this notoriety. The media like all this, they like me, whether it is good, bad or ugly, so it's about time that I made it work for me."

It was as if a little light had been switched on in my brain. I woke up to the fact that all the plastic surgery I'd had made me newsworthy, so I decided that I was going to see if I could cash in on it.

But before that, something wonderful happened to me. Tony asked me to marry him, of course I said yes, and in September 2005 we finally got hitched. What a fantastic day.

Most women go on diets before their wedding day, but I visited the plastic surgeon for a facelift. I had made up my mind that my marriage to Tony would be the last time I walked down the aisle, and I wanted to look my very best for him, so what better way?

The procedure lasted about 40 minutes – only slightly longer than it took us to get married actually. I recovered quickly, with no bruising and very little swelling – even I have to admit that I am very fortunate in this respect. Some women go through all sorts of agony, but not me. I also had a breast uplift and some liposuction.

Truth be told, the day after the surgery I took myself off shopping.

When I had my breasts uplifted, the surgeon actually removed the nipples, reattaching them only when he had got everything else neatly back in place. And so I had two pert new boobs. And very nice they looked too. I knew that Tony would be as pleased with them as I was. The best thing of all was I could now walk around without a bra and my puppies both remained in place, exactly as God intended.

So when our wedding day arrived, I thought that I looked pretty good, and so did Tony. I have no hesitation in saying that it turned out to be the best wedding day of my life, and I have had more practice than most.

Tony had gone to stay in a hotel the night before. It was nothing to do with tradition – he just didn't want to be in a house full of women.

In true Barbie fashion, there was lots of pink. As I have already said, my wedding to John was a pretty low-key affair, and I was determined that this was going to be the one of my dreams, so we had a marquee that was filled with pink flowers, ribbons, balloons and pink hearts. It sat beside a lake and there were even swans gently gliding across the water.

The weather was fantastic, the food was great, and we had superb music supplied by a Latin band and a disco. It was like a fairytale.

We got married at 5pm – I know that many people would consider that to be late in the day, but I needed the time to get ready. For this marriage, I had really made an effort. Having decided to live up to the Barbie image, I wore a pink wedding gown with shocking pink veil, which had been custom-made in Italy.

I arrived at Cambridge register office with my six bridesmaids, including Charlotte, Hannah and Poppy, and I felt on top of the world. Naturally, the girls were all dressed in pink too. All day long I had listened to the birds singing, and everything felt perfect.

As I walked down the aisle, Tony turned to look at me and there were tears in his eyes. When I reached him, he whispered: "It's about bloody time. You look amazing."

My mother recited a poem and then we waited with baited breath when the registrar asked if there was anybody present who knew of any reason why our wedding should not go ahead. And then I heard I waited so long to hear: "I now pronounce you man and wife. You may kiss the bride."

And Tony did, a long, lingering kiss that compounded my joy.

Then it was back to the marquee, where Dad's speech referred to the night he dragged me, kicking and screaming out of the disco all those years ago after I had lied about Tony's parents being away for the weekend. "Needless to say, the journey home was silent," he said.

Then my mother, who has always had a fabulous voice, sang *Love Me Tender*. It was a glorious day that turned into an unforgettable night, with everybody keeping the speeches short and getting the tone just right.

It was only sad that my brother Trevor and Tony's father, Ted, couldn't have been there to see me come full circle and finally marry the man I was destined to spend the rest of my life with.

CHAPTER 17
Welcome To My World

Dozens of messages had been left on my answering machine, and business cards and suchlike had been pushed through the letterbox by journalists who wanted my story, so I started to call them back, but this was going to be done on my terms, so the first question I asked was: "Come on, what's in it for me?"

If they were going to sell newspapers based on what I was going to tell them, then I wanted a part of the action. It seemed to me that everybody else was doing it, so why not me?

Even back then you couldn't pick up a newspaper or magazine without reading about what Katie Price and Kerry Katona were up to, and they weren't giving their stories away for nothing.

To be honest, I wasn't sure whether I could pull this one off, but I decided to give it a damn good try. As long as you give something your best shot, that's all you can ask.

I started off my appearing on the *Lorraine Kelly Show*, but only on condition that the benefit fraud wasn't brought up. They agreed. I have to say that it was all a bit of a disaster because I was so nervous. In fact, I was properly scared. I hadn't done anything like this before and when they said that they wanted me to talk like an air-headed bimbo it wasn't difficult. I wasn't properly prepared, and I had no idea how long they wanted me to speak or how to interact with the camera. And once I got started, I wouldn't let Lorraine get a word in, which didn't exactly endear me to her.

At the end of the show, she walked off without talking to me, so I guess that I must have upset her. She forgot that this was my first time, and I would have thought it would have been in her best interests to have spoken to me beforehand and to tell me what she expected, so my view was that she got what she deserved.

But I was off and running. Next came *The Mirror* and they branded me 'The £100,000 Real-Life Barbie' on account of all the plastic surgery. They paid me about £5,000 for talking to them, and they also gave me the name that has stuck with me, and for that I owe them a debt of gratitude because I was more than happy to go away and develop and play up to this image.

The picture that appeared in *The Mirror's* double-page spread was of me wearing a really short dress, and I loved both the photo and the article.

Once again, the phone started ringing off the hook. Newspapers, television and radio producers all wanted to talk to me. As I was fielding all these inquiries, I suddenly realised: "Sarah, you are going to make a living out of this, girl. You are going to make a living out of just being who you are and telling people what you have done and what you have had done to your body." I couldn't believe it. Why hadn't I thought of this myself? Sometimes, the best things come along when you least expect them.

I should say one thing before I go any further. Growing up, I hated Barbie. I always preferred playing with Action Man and with real boys. I was never into dolls, but here I was, in my forties, being given a new identity, and a fresh start. And boy, did I feel that I deserved a fresh start. It was also really important to me that I start contributing financially after everything that Tony had done for me. He had never once complained, but things were very difficult for him.

"Okay, I don't really like being branded Barbie, but the media seem to like it so let's play along with it and see where it takes us," I thought. So I bought myself a website and called it www.reallifebarbie.com and packed it with information about myself, along with plenty of glamorous images.

It continues to go from strength to strength and I know that if you are sufficiently interested then you will log on for yourself, but here is a flavour of what appears on the home page:

She's British upper class, outspoken, demanding, gorgeously wacky and totally plastic apart from the boobs (always armed with a syringe of filler in one hand and a glass of champagne in the other). She has appeared on TV and radio around the world and is a strong contender or having had the most cosmetic procedures and now she's boarding a plane to the USA.

In the UK she's been seen, heard and read about on morning TV and radio's most popular programmes. Sarah's a familiar face on such programmes as GMTV, This Morning, and the BBC as well as a variety of prime-time terrestrial TV programmes such as Celebrity Ding Dong, The Big Question and loads more. She has become a cult figure in Japan after her 'Life as Barbie' docudrama was broadcast to 14 million viewers on Nippon TV – her increasing popularity has spread throughout Japan's porn industry who asked if she would make porn movies with them! How fabulous is that! And now she needs bodyguards to hold back the crowds when she visits Japan!

Sarah B, the gorgeously wacky living Barbie doll, has careered, dressed and impressed her way through life. Just like Barbie, she can be anything you want her to be!

Millions of men and women around the world are unhappy with their lives, bodies and environment. Sarah was among them. She grabbed life with both hands and changed from being an 'average looking' housewife into 'sex on *legs' and wowing the world by undergoing $1m of plastic surgery! She is a completely different person, beaming with self confidence and character! She has given herself a new lease of life and now she's ready for some serious action and being Sooo Naughty!*

As you will have gathered from that extract, it was never meant to be taken seriously, but the whole thing just snowballed. I had nothing in common with Barbie apart from the name I had been given by *The Mirror*, but it worked.

I became a Media Motormouth. If ever they wanted an example of somebody who'd undergone lots of plastic surgery, they came to me for pictures; and if ever they wanted a view from somebody about the advantages, and disadvantages, of plastic surgery they came to me for a quote.

I guess the Internet became my biggest friend. What surprised me most of all was that the interest in me was from all over the world, and that can only have been because of my website and things that had been said and written about me on the net. I found myself in television studios in London talking to audiences in countries such as Australia and Japan; I appeared in magazine articles in Singapore and India; I was flown out to America, Poland, Greece and Germany.

And, bizarrely, I would find myself sitting in a satellite studio with an interpreter by my side if I was appearing in a country where they did not speak English. The strangest of those was when I was asked if I would appear on a Russian television programme. There was an interpreter beside me in London and another in the studio in Moscow, and although I couldn't see the studio audience, I was told that members of The Anti-Barbie Movement were present. What? Barbie is a doll. What is there not to like about a doll? Or was the protest against me?

No, the protest was against Barbie, the doll. They thought it created a bad image for children. I cannot understand why young girls would not aspire to have long blonde hair and look beautiful, but what do I know?

Funny people, the Russians. It was very difficult to take that one seriously. The other thing, of course, is that you have to sit there and pray that the interpreter is giving a faithful and accurate translation of what you have said. I never had any way of knowing, and still don't. But you get a feeling from the way the audience reacts.

I would sit down for an interview and a journalist would ask why I had surgery to make myself look like Barbie. Okay, if that was what they wanted to hear, that is what I would give them. I was quite capable of spinning out any angle they wanted, and the more I did it, the better I became at playing the game. In the end, they were writing the stories I wanted them to write, but they were the ones who thought that they were controlling me.

And the more that was written about me, the more they wanted.

Eventually I realised that I had to get myself an agent to deal with all the inquiries because there was so much work coming in, although I resented having hand over a percentage of my earnings, so that relationship did not last long. Next, I employed a PR company, but I was so busy that they came to me and told me they couldn't cope with all the work.

Tony and I came to the conclusion that it was best for the two of us to handle everything ourselves, and he ended up giving up most of his business interests so that he could work with me and make sure that everything ticked along as it should do. As our business relationship developed, so he became my manager.

Tony had bought his ex-wife a house, not far from where we live. On top of that, he was paying her maintenance. As you can imagine, it was terribly difficult for him financially and then with the economic squeeze, he lost his company as well.

He acted as a middle man, sourcing aluminium at the best possible price and then supplying it, but in times of recession, people always find a way of cutting out the middle man. The final straw was when a couple of firms that owed him something in region of £150,000 went bust. These things always have a knock-on effect. Going bust himself was the only option left to Tony.

With that, he had to stop the maintenance payments and he asked his ex to give him a couple of months to get back on his feet and he would see her right. That is one thing with Tony – he always bounces back. Another is that if he says he is going to do something, he will always do it, and that included the payments to Rebecca.

But she wouldn't have any of it and before we knew where we were, Tony was in court, where he was ordered to pay £7,000 in back payments as well as £600 a month. "But at this moment, I don't have it, so where is it going to come from?" he asked. By this time, Tony and I were married, so he was told that he would have to get the money from me.

You will not be hugely surprised to learn that I refused. Why would I want to give her a penny of my hard-earned money? She hadn't done too badly out of Tony when all was said and done – she'd got a house and a car, and if she'd only had a little patience and faith, the payments would have resumed before long. It wasn't as if she was destitute – apart form anything else, she had a boyfriend with whom she'd had a baby.

What happened next? Another court case. It was made clear that if the money wasn't paid, there was a very real chance of Tony being sent to prison until it was paid, so I had no choice. Before long, we were virtually on our knees. Tony had a Jaguar. It was his pride and joy, a reward for all the hard work he had done over the years, and we had to hide it because he was afraid it would be seized. It was another dreadful period.

Eventually we went to the Child Support Agency and asked them to step in – it was the only way we could think of to protect my earnings because although the Magistrates' Courts had the power to order me to pay his ex, the CSA couldn't. It still wasn't pretty, but at least it meant we were able to keep hold of something.

I was affected by the recession too. The newspapers and television still wanted to talk to me, but they were no longer paying me as much, so I was depending more and more upon work coming in from abroad.

This was the new Sarah though, and I wasn't down for too long. Next up was HumanHi. This merits some explanation. It is all about the buzz you get when you reach your fulfilment – that could be taking part in your first skydive, or it could be about the feeling that you get when you qualify to become a doctor. It might be the emotion a runner gets when he crosses the finishing line having completed his first marathon, of the way a parent feels when a baby son or daughter takes his or her first steps.

Of course, it stands for 'Human High', but in this computer age, we abbreviated it to HumanHi. All my life I have been striving to find my ultimate high. I have always been ambitious...

And so I set up www.humanhi.com and it is a place people can go to share their dreams and ambitions with other like-minded individuals. My HumanHi was, of course, getting to where I am in my life now with Tony and Poppy, and then discovering this strange quirk of fate, that the very thing that had landed me in court was the same thing that could help to turn my life around and help me to earn a living. It wasn't planned. Very few of the things I have done in my life have been planned – things just have a habit of happening to me, and I go along for the ride and see where it takes me.

But every person knows when they have reached a stage of fulfilment in their lives – the key thing is to embrace it and make the most of it when it happens to you because it could be snatched away in an instant.

I turned my infamy into a positive, and that was my HumanHi, and, just like Real-Life Barbie, it has been picked up on all around the world, with an American television company approaching me and asking me to front a programme that explored the journeys certain people take to find fulfilment.

My life has been an adventure and although I have met some wicked people who were interested only in seeing what they could get out of me, and then throwing me away when they had finished with me, I have always met some absolutely amazing individuals.

When I have come a cropper in my life, there have always been one or two individuals who have been there for me, people who wanted to help and expected nothing in return.

One such person is a man called Martin Marshall, who is a photographer and film-maker. He is a brilliant man, and I first came across him when I was doing some work on plastic surgery for local television. Originally, Martin was a media lawyer, who lives in Norfolk, and he contacted the television studio and expressed an interested in getting in touch with me because he said that he wanted to document my life.

He told them that he was convinced that there was more to me than being a walking advertisement for plastic surgery. We were eventually put in contact with another and he came to Cambridgeshire to meet me – it goes without saying that I was wary of him. He was a complete stranger, after all. But sometimes you have to take chances, and I have always believed it is important that if you get a good immediate gut feeling about somebody then you should go with that feeling.

I made sure that Tony was with me, and the two of us settled down and listened to what he had to say. In effect, he was proposing that he make a documentary about my life. He stressed that if this was something I wanted to do, I should not allow a television company to do it because I would lose control and they could edit things as they saw fit.

He promised that I would see everything and that I would have to be happy with the content before he would try and market it.

I explained to him that one of the problems was that Faisal had destroyed all my family photographs and videos, which meant that there was nothing showing me running around in the garden with my brother or with my parents. "It doesn't matter Sarah," he said. "As a film-maker, I can go into the archives and drag out pictures and footage of the 1960s and 1970s and recreate the atmosphere for you – it will not be your friends and family, but it will still be part of your story. But the best thing would be if you had a book, an autobiography, something that tells your life story. I can then bring those pages to life."

I was transfixed by everything he said, right up to the point where he suggested that I write a book.

"Martin, I can't write a book," I told him. "I am not a writer. You write it for me."

"I can't do that. I am a film-maker, not a writer. Trust me Sarah, your life story deserves to be put down for posterity in a book."

"But I wouldn't know where to begin."

"You just think about all the things that have happened in your life, and you go back to the start and you put it down on paper. Just think about what you have been through."

It got me thinking. Maybe he was correct after all. But it was the start of a friendship, and one of the reasons it has been such a strong friendship is because he never wanted anything back. Martin has always been happy just to be a friend, somebody to have a bit of a laugh and a joke with.

So the seed had been planted in my mind and then, right out of the blue, I was approached by a London publisher who had read all about me in various tabloid newspaper and followed up with some research of his own on the Internet, and he asked me to go and meet him.

Once more, I was full of hope and optimism. Will I never learn? The truth is that I hadn't a clue what 'being published' meant or involved. Despite my conversations with Martin, I really hadn't the foggiest idea how to go about writing my life story. What would people be interested in reading? And if I thought something was exciting or funny, would that mean the man or woman in the street would do too?

As I sat in front of this publisher he asked me: "So Sarah, what ideas have you got for your book?"

I sat in front of him like a dummy. "I haven't a clue. Remember that it was you who asked me to come and see you."

"Yes, but I hoped that you might have given this matter some thought."

"I have thought of little else, but I am not a writer."

He told me about various books that had been written by people who were not obvious celebrities, and suggested that I go and read one or two of them. And he got my attention when he told me that these were books that had made decent sums of money for the individuals involved.

"Do you see it being packed with colour pictures?"

I didn't know.

"Have you written anything at all?"

I hadn't written a single word, and I was made to feel that I was wasting this man's time, despite the fact that he was the one who had approached me, and he was the one who had asked me to come to his office. Had he asked me to put down a few ideas, I would have done so, but he caught me cold. I felt like a fish out of water. This whole world of publishing was completely alien to me and I knew that I had looked like a blithering idiot who was incapable of stringing more than a couple of words together.

I asked him what he wanted from me and he told me to go away and write a couple of sample chapters. It was easy enough for him to say that but I barely had to write the shopping list because that was something Tony did, and it is something all my previous partners had done.

And how on earth do you write a 'sample chapter' of your life? What would a publisher be looking for? Would he want to read a 'sample chapter' about me being beaten to within an inch of my life? Would he want to read a 'sample chapter' about my sexual experiments with a spoon and a teenage friend? Would he want to read a 'sample chapter' about me having sex with a Hollywood legend? Would he want to read a 'sample chapter' about Michael Rutt?

I thought about nothing else for about a week and one morning I woke up at about 5am and went straight to the computer and started writing. And I didn't stop until I had finished. In the meantime, I didn't eat properly, I hardly slept or washed. When I did go to bed, I had a pen and paper by my bedside so that when I woke up and remembered things – and I did, almost every night – I could make a note of it before I forgot it.

Trust me, I got properly into character, living the Bohemian lifestyle to the full, and my family knew not to disturb me. Night and day. Day and night. And then, after three solid months, I had finished it.

Remember I spoke earlier about HumanHi? This was a HumanHi, a moment of fulfilment. I had written my autobiography. In my ignorance, I thought that all I had to do was send it off to the publisher, he would turn it into a nice hardback book and in no time at all I would have a best-seller on my hands. Get the sports car ordered, and the luxury foreign holiday...

So I put the words into an email attachment and I sent it off to the publisher. I expected him to come back to me almost immediately and sign me up to this fabulous deal, but days went by and I hadn't heard a word. What I didn't realise was that he had to read the manuscript and assess it himself, and then seek the opinions of the various people in his marketing and sales departments, many of whom would, of course, be women. I could be way, way off beam here, but I have always believed that my story would alienate just as many women as it would attract – I had abandoned my daughter, and that was bad enough. But I had also put myself under the knife, and for a lot of women, that was ever worse. Just let them go through the beatings I was subjected to and then see if they change their minds.

I was champing at the bit. I had given up three months of my life, and I wanted this publisher to come back to me yesterday with an answer. I expected him to drop everything for me.

When he did get back to me, it wasn't with the words I was expecting to hear. "Hi Sarah. Well, I have read your manuscript, I really enjoyed it, there is so much gripping stuff in there and I think you have the makings of a fabulous autobiography [those were the words I was expecting to hear] but..."

Why is there always a 'but'?

"But my sales team have convinced me that your profile is not sufficiently high for your book to sell in significant numbers, so I am afraid that I cannot offer you a publishing deal after all. I am really sorry."

Not half as sorry as I was. "I see, so it's back to the theatre school days of being the nearly girl, is it? Getting so close and then being given the big heave-ho." I was devastated, but I always believed that some day, somebody would publish it. After sitting down and producing a manuscript I knew that Martin had been right all along and that I did have a brilliant story to tell; even I couldn't believe some of it.

I have never been one to rest on my laurels and, as you will discover, the offers just kept coming, but they did not always take me in the direction I had hoped to go with them. Not only that, but there were to be more bitter disappointments and some poor judgement calls by yours truly.

I have always made good reportage but now, at the age of 45, I had launched a career.

CHAPTER 18
Under The Knife

I have touched upon it throughout, but now is the moment of truth, when I tell you all about my plastic surgery. It began for me when I was just seven years old – like many children, I had been born with an ear that stuck out.

Girls are lucky because they can let their hair grow and it hides things like that, but I became pretty self-conscious of something that I regarded as a deformity and I pestered my parents until my mother took me to see the doctor, who agreed to refer me to a specialist at Great Ormond Street Hospital and finally my right ear was pinned back. I remember having the anaesthetic and enjoying the experience.

I wasn't at all nervous about any of it – in fact, I went out of my way to read up about the procedure that was going to be involved. The best bit was that, although I knew there might be some pain, the doctor was going to fix my ear and make me look normal, like all my friends.

Today, a child who'd had his or her ears pinned back would probably be sent home the same day, but I was kept in for a couple of days and, being the precocious child that I was, I took it upon myself to entertain the other children, some of whom were quite poorly. I would sing songs and read them stories.

I had a hand mirror on my bedside table, and the moment I came around I started fumbling for it because I wanted to see the result of the surgery. What I hadn't realised was that my head would be covered in bandages – I had expected to be able to inspect the surgeon's handiwork immediately, and I was quite disappointed that I couldn't.

"Where's my new ear? Can we take this off so that I can have a look at it?" And I was about to start undoing everything until a nurse explained in no uncertain terms that I mustn't. I wanted to be repaired immediately so that I could move on with my life.

I was at home for bonfire night, but still had the bandage on my head, so I had to watch the fireworks from my bedroom window, which I hated.

And then came the day of the big reveal. When my bandages were finally removed I was very impressed with the result, even as a child, and I guess you could say that I was bitten by the bug way back then. I was hugely confident all of a sudden, and wanted to start wearing my hair up and behind my ears. It quite literally transformed me.

My appearance was never an issue for me until I saw the photos of my second wedding, to Glenn. I was 26 and I realised, with horror, that I had a bit of a double chin. At 26! It had to go.

People tried to tell me that it was puppy fat, but it wasn't. This was proper fat, set in for life and there was no way it was going away of its own volition.

I got hold of a copy of *Yellow Pages*, flicked through, picked a clinic in Watford of all places, made the phone call, arranged the appointment and turned up to have it done.

"So, will you be using a local anaesthetic?"

"Don't you worry about that my dear. We will just suck that fat straight out and you will be as good as new."

I insisted that I wanted them to numb my chin, and they did. Ten minutes later it was done and as they started to put the bandages on I said: "You can't do that. I can't get on a train home looking like that."

They insisted that it should remain on, but I took it off, got on the train and went home. Job done. Good God! How naïve was I?

Not only had I done no checks on this clinic, meaning that I didn't even know if the person who performed the procedure was even fit and able to do so, but I hadn't really checked out the procedure itself. All that I knew was that I had developed a double chin and I wanted rid of it.. The surgeon, who was a woman, could have been a voodoo witch doctor for all I knew, or a butcher.

Luck played a huge part. I felt no pain, and as the days went by so I began to notice an improvement until eventually, when all the swelling had gone down, I realised that my double chin, or puppy fat, had vanished into the ether.

Plastic surgery? Cosmetic procedures? A walk in the park! And it only cost me about £600.

Then I started to notice the crow's feet around my eyes. If only I had the money, I could transform my appearance.

I had seen the benefits of one procedure and that is when I became obsessive about the whole thing. Even at that stage, I began to draw up a wish list of things that I could have done. Obviously, all of this was before I had been beaten to a pulp, and I am the first to admit that way back then it was all about vanity, whereas eventually my obsession would be driven by necessity, by a desire to put right what had been taken away from me.

The plastic surgery began for real after I'd had my looks rearranged. Let me state here and now that I have no issues with the National Health Service. They were interested only in getting me better and getting me home and, without the care I received, I dread to think what would have happened.

But, to be frank, they were not interested in how I looked, only in making sure that everything worked. I felt like a patchwork quilt, like they had taken bits and pieces of various people and stuck them all together on my face and body, and nothing looked any good. And I was desperately unhappy with my nose in particular. This was no fault of the NHS – it had been broken, just like a boxer's, and it bore no resemblance to the one I had been born with. I hated many parts of my appearance during this stage of my life, but nothing more so than my nose.

I pleaded and pleaded with my doctor and he arranged for me to see a plastic surgeon who eventually agreed to remodel it for me. It is worth explaining that when you go to see a Harley Street plastic surgeon for a nose job, you are asked what sort of nose you want – you tell the surgeon, and he will inform you whether or not he will be able to do it. If you are paying the money, you usually get pretty much exactly what you want.

It is not like that with the NHS. Yes, the doctor agreed that my nose was pretty badly distorted, and he promised to do everything that he could to put it right. The surgeon knew what had happened to me, and he realised how depressed I was about the way I looked.

He told me that he knew how I should look, so I trusted him totally and agreed to let him operate on my nose. Perhaps I should have asked more questions, but maybe I didn't want to hear the answers.

In the lead-up to the operations, all my meetings had been with the consultant, but I didn't realise at the time that he would not be performing my operation – it was to be done by his registrar. The operation took place in the NHS hospital in Rickmansworth and as far as I was concerned, everything had gone to plan.

I was sent home, swathed in bandages and a plaster that I had to keep on for two or three weeks. Then I had to go back for the great unveiling.

"Go on Sarah, take a look, I am certain you will be delighted with what we've done..." The bandages had been removed from my face and the nurse thrust a mirror into my hand, urging me to look at the surgeon's handiwork.

I was so horrified by what had been done to me that I fainted. If anything, they had made things worse, and that was even allowing for the fact that I knew there would still be some swelling that had to settle down.

By now, the registrar was in the room, and he was obviously concerned about what had happened. My words to him were something like: "Is it going to change? Please tell me this is not as good as it is going to get. It is going to settle down, isn't it, please tell me it is."

"Well you are very bruised here and here," he said pointing to various areas of my nose, "and it will settle down to an extent."

I was in floods of tears. What had I done to deserve this? Was I being paid back for all the terrible things that I done in my life? Why had I been made to look even more hideous now than I was before? It just wasn't fair. How much worse could my life get?

The doctor didn't know what to say or do. As far as he was concerned, everything was all right, and he had done as he had been asked.

I cannot tell you much I hated my nose. I had been unhappy with it before, but the thought that this was as good as it was ever going to be filled me with horror, and I didn't want anybody to see me. The best thing was just to lock myself away because nobody, surely, would want to look at me. It may not have been as bad as all that, but the bottom line was that I hated it, and that was all that mattered.

It wasn't what I had asked for, and it wasn't what I expected, so I went back to see the consultant and told him how I felt. Imagine my horror when he said that he wouldn't be able to do anything for at least another two years. Then I went back to my own doctor and all that he wanted to do was to send me to see a psychiatrist. None of this was helping me.

There was nothing for it but to soldier on because at that stage in my life I couldn't afford to have private treatment, and I sure as hell wasn't going to put myself in the hands of the NHS again, not when they couldn't see what an awful job they'd done.

It wasn't until I was in my thirties that I finally found my own way to Harley Street and started to link up with plastic surgeons through having my own space in their consulting rooms. And boy, did I ever make up for lost time.

Before long, it reached the stage where I was having operations done almost as job lots. My first priority, naturally, was to have my nose fixed once and for all. At the same time that was being done, I also had chin implants. I was a woman on a mission, and I was a woman in a hurry.

I knew that I was in the hands of the men who were the best in Britain, and possibly the world, at what they did. And it was in their interests to do it properly – if I was going to be a walking advertisement for their skills and abilities, obviously they would want to get it right, so I felt that I couldn't possibly lose.

The consultant I had seen on the NHS was a chap called Douglas Harrison, who insisted that he felt his registrar had done a good job on my nose. I told him he was just saying that because he felt that he had to, and when he realised that I wasn't going to take no for an answer, he agreed to give me the nose job I wanted.

He performed the operation for me at the Bishops Wood Hospital. It should have taken no longer than 90 minutes, but it actually lasted more than four hours. Mr Harrison later admitted that he couldn't believe the mess he found when he opened up my nose – not because the registrar had botched the first operation, but because my nose had taken such a terrible beating when I was attacked.

And that was why the registrar had found it so difficult to give me the nose I wanted. But Douglas Harrison managed it after taking bits of cartilage from my ear.

This time, when the bandages and plaster came off I was happy with what I saw in the mirror. Some six years had gone by since my NHS operation, six years during which I cringed every time I looked in a mirror. But no longer.

My obsession was to put right all the things that were wrong with me – all the things that had been broken or damaged. So there were chin implants that hid the after-effects of my broken jaw; and there were cheek implants, which helped to fill out the dents where my cheekbone and eye socket had been broken.

Mr Harrison was responsible for those procedures, too. The guy is a genius.

It was an empowering experience, and it transformed my life. Before the plastic surgery began, I would get up every day and know that I would have to look at my face in the mirror before I applied the make-up that would at least make me look presentable to the world. And every single morning, I would relive, to some degree or other, that night when I thought that I was going to die.

But now, those memories were beginning to fade and I was once more becoming the woman I wanted to be.

I need to stress again how important it was for me to look the part. I was helping women to improve their appearance and I was recommending specific plastic surgeons to them, so they had to be able to look at me and be happy with what they saw. If they realised that not only had I had these procedures done myself, but that they had been successful, then there was a far greater chance that they would use the surgeon I was recommending. And if that happened, then everybody would be happy.

The implants caused my skin to become dimpled, so next on the agenda was laser treatment for my face. People don't realise, but it is quite common for one solution to cause another problem, which then has to be addressed, so I always tell anybody who is thinking of having plastic surgery to do as much research as possible and, always, to ask questions, no matter how stupid you may think they are.

It also helps to explain, I believe, why people become addicted – they have one thing done and realise it means that they have to get something else done as a consequence. And when that has been done, there is always something else. Always. I suppose it is a bit like those poor men who paint the Forth Bridge – no sooner have they got to the end than they have to cross back over the River Forth and start all over again. And, of course, the effects of many procedures are temporary, so you have to keep "topping up".

Lots of women have breast implants fitted and after a while they go rock solid – first of all, the skin dimples up and looks extremely unattractive, and then they have to be replaced – mind you, that is far preferable to have an implant burst inside your body. There are countless stories of women being poisoned through silicon leaking into their bloodstream, and some have suffered agonising deaths as a result. It simply reinforces how incredibly dangerous cosmetic surgery can be, and how important it is to find a reputable surgeon, somebody who puts his patients' well-being before his profit margin.

Uniquely, I actually had my breasts reduced, and I am proud to say that, even now, they are entirely natural. There are no implants, or anything else floating around inside my tits that do not belong to me, that I was not born with. I have had them uplifted, but only because gravity eventually took its toll.

It's about the only part of my body that is my own, even though people often accuse me of having had a breast enlargement. Trust me – the boobs God gave me were too big! Objects of joy and delight for many of the men in my life, obviously, but bloody uncomfortable for me.

People talk about experiencing pain and discomfort when they undergo cosmetic surgery, especially with any procedure that involves the face, but I never felt anything – perhaps, once again, it goes back to being beaten up. I could apply skin peels and although my face would be red raw, I felt nothing.

Most women have anaesthetic when they have fillers and botox applied to their face – not me. Put me in a dentist's chair, however, and I am climbing the walls. I hate it. I can't even stand going to see the hygienist. All the scraping – it's just horrible.

After I had Charlotte, I was left with stretch marks. There is nothing you can about that, it's just one of those things. You will not be surprised to learn that I didn't like it, but I learnt to live with it, and I wore clothes that hid it – even when I had to wear swimsuits and bikinis, if you are clever you can disguise no end of things, including stretch marks.

After I gave birth to Poppy following a caesarean section, I decided that it was time the stretch marks went too, so I had a tummy tuck. I was told that the result would not be perfect, but if it meant getting rid of the scar and most of the stretch marks, then it seemed like a pretty good outcome to me. While the surgeon was doing that he also did buttock implants.

Operating on the front and back at the same time is pretty much unheard of, and the surgeon told me he didn't really want to do it.

"What do you mean? Why don't you want to do it? I am not having my tummy done, waiting for it to heal and then coming back again to have my bum done. Go on – do it in one go. I will be absolutely fine. Oh, and while you are at it, do my eyes, liposuction and fat transfer."

"I know you are a tough cookie," he said. "But you are talking about five procedures in one go, and that breaks all boundaries. I don't think you realise quite what you are asking me to do. You will not be able to stand the pain, I promise you."

"Don't you worry about my pain barriers. Once you have done it, I will just have to hack it. You can always say, 'I told you so', but I really do want all of this done in one hit.

Reluctantly, he agreed. And let me clear something up right now. You will remember that the article that landed me in hot water with the DSS was the one in which I had talked about a bum implant – the article appeared in 2005, but I didn't have the damn procedure carried out until 2007.

He started off working on my stomach, then when he had done that he stitched me up, turned me over, sliced open my backside, dropped in the inserts, stitched that up, turned me over again and then did my eyes and the liposuction. And I had told him to insert the fat in my hands to make them look younger.

Where he did draw the line was with the anaesthetic – I asked him to give me a local, but he informed me that the pain would probably kill me, so I let him have his way on that one. I was on the operating table for about five hours and when I came round there were tubes sticking out of various parts of my body, but I felt absolutely fine and told the surgeon that I wanted to go home.

"Go home? Are you mad, Sarah? You need to stay in for two days at the very least, and then we will see how you are."

I wasn't having any of that – the advantage of having had as many operations and procedures as I have is that you quickly get to know your own body, what it will take, what you as an individual can take. In the end, we compromised and I stayed in overnight and returned home the next day, leaving him shaking his head it utter disbelief.

Admittedly, there was some degree of discomfort. For a start, I couldn't sleep on my back and I couldn't sleep on my front, because I had been operated upon on both sides.

And then the pain hit. I have never experienced anything like it and don't mind admitting that it reduced me to tears. I was in agony. I lay in bed and complained to Tony about how sore my bum was, but he wasn't particularly sympathetic, pointing out that it had been my choice, and that it had been me who had insisted upon having everything done in one go. Oh, how I regretted it.

"You put yourself through it, you vain cow. You have nobody to blame but yourself. Nobody forced you, and the doctor did advise you against it," Tony said.

"I know, I know, but you are going to have to see to Poppy. Leave me alone, I just want to die."

"Okay, I will do it. Just get better, and quickly."

Then I had a problem with the wound from the tummy tuck, which started seeping. I thought I was in trouble – it is never a good sign when that sort of thing happens. I knew that I had to go back to the hospital and get the wound re-dressed. Fortunately, there was nothing wrong with the surgery, and it just turned out to be one of those things, which they sorted out for me immediately.

On the way home, I had to tell Tony to stop the car because the pain I was experiencing from my bum was beyond description. Why hadn't I listened to the doctor in the first place? Why couldn't I have been patient and had these things done one at a time, like any normal person?

I also knew that if I should have been experiencing extreme pain anywhere, it should have been from my tummy, not from my bottom. In the end, I decided to grin and bear it, and after about a week the pain finally went away.

There has been a side-effect that I have had to learn to live with. Many people get water on the knee, but since I have had my bum implants fitted, from time to time I get a fluid build-up in one buttock or the other – never both at the same time. It means that one buttock becomes bigger than the other one. Fortunately, it doesn't last for long, so it is something I have learnt to live with and to laugh at. The surgeon has told me he can removed the implants and replace them but there are no guarantees that the same thing will not happen again, so it is just something I have to live with.

An added complication was and is the fact that if he did take them out, it would be six months before they could be replaced. No way.

I have been asked where I draw the line, whether there are any procedures I would not have done. There is a process which is commonly available in Japan for people who want to be taller – it involves breaking the patient's legs and attaching inserts. I cannot imagine anything worse, and I would never consider something like that. To have something like that done as a cosmetic procedure is insane.

My appearance is important to me – let's face it, without looking the way I do, and without having gone through all these operations, I would not have a career. That means I see cosmetic surgery as part of an ongoing maintenance programme, and I have no plans to quit any time soon.

Fortunately, I have put myself in good hands and been operated on by the best in the business, and as long as I think they keep me looking good – and youthful – why on earth would I want to stop?

I regard myself as an ambassador for good plastic surgery. My God, there are some awful cosmetic surgeons out there, and there are people who simply don't know where to draw the line. America is the worst – it seems that just about everybody you meet looks as if they have just climbed off the back of a motorbike. They look completely unnatural and in many, many cases they cannot even manage a smile because of all the work they have had done on their faces.

Perhaps the most extreme case is that of Jocelyn Wildenstein who, after divorcing her multi-millionaire husband, spent more than £2m on assorted procedures and has now been dubbed 'The Bride Of Wildenstein'. I believe that the surgeons who continued to operate upon this poor woman should be ashamed of themselves – was it really so important for them to make money that they would carry on without a thought as to the result of their work?

Wildenstein looks like a monster. Just check out the Internet and then tell me I am wrong. While I am a fan of plastic surgery, it is blatantly obvious that it is does need to be regulated and that in various parts of the world there are some unscrupulous individuals who have no interest in the welfare of the women (and men) upon whom they operate. These individuals have no right to be called cosmetic surgeons, and should be struck off. It worries me, even now, that the industry is not sufficiently well regulated.

And if somebody makes a hideous mess of your face, there is not an awful lot you can do about it. I have people tell me that if I carry on, I will end up looking like Michael Jackson. I beg your pardon? I know what I am doing – more important than that, the people who operate on me know what they are doing.

When I refer people, I send them to the right man for the job. I don't pack them off willy-nilly because that would be both irresponsible and dangerous. When I recommend a cosmetic surgeon for a specific procedure it is because I know that he is the best at that procedure, not some voodoo doctor.

The law of averages suggests that every time I have something done so the risk that something will go wrong increases, but I am happy to put myself in the hands of these wonderful men. As things stand right now, I intend to carry on having cosmetic surgery for as long as I am physically able to do so.

Everybody always wants to know how much my plastic surgery has cost. If I had forked out for it all myself, these are the bills I would have had to pay:

FACE:

Whole face lasered to remove layer of skin to give a youthful look – four times, every five years, cost £32,000;

Gortex filler threaded into frown lines around nose and mouth to remove lines, £5,000;

Dermabrasion to entire face every five years – a procedure where skin is sanded to remove the top layer, makes the face look younger, £20,000;

Facelift - a half inch cut was made in front of each ear, the skin over the face pulled tight then sown back to the front of the ear, £6,500;

Second facelift as one side looked lop-sided, so a similar nip-tuck was carried out, £6,500;

Another facelift plus upper eyes four years later, £13,500;

More gortex filler threaded through facial lines following facelift, £5,000;

Endoscopic brow lift, £12,000;

Fat transfer to hands, cheeks, lips, chin, hollow of eyes, £6,000;

Solid silicone implant fed into each cheek through the mouth to avoid scars on the face, £7,000;

Liposuction to chin and neck, fat sucked out through a catheter-type tube, £4,000;

Silicone implant was again fed through the mouth, £6,500;

Replacement implant to resume asymmetry following facelifts, £7,500;

Liposuction to jaw bi-yearly for the last 20 years, £30,000;

Upper lip and surrounding areas, dermabrasion bi-yearly for last 20 years to prevent lines, £35,000;

Upper eye lift, excess skin was cut out from the lid and folds stitched together, £5,500;

Lower eye area lasered to get rid of wrinkles, £4,000;

Lower eyes lasered again, £4,000

Nose job £5,000;

Second nose job, £8,500;

Ear pinned back, £7,000.

TEETH:

Laser treatment x four, every five years, £18,000.

BREASTS:

Reduction from a 32H 32DD. Nipples were removed and sewn on again and flesh folded and liposuction to each side, £12,000;

Breast uplift, £6,500;

Second uplift, £8,000.

STOMACH:

Liposuction to remove excess skin that could not be shifted in the gym, £4,500;

Tummy tuck, £7,500;

More liposuction to stomach following tummy tuck as it wasn't flat enough, £3,000.

HIPS:

Liposuction to hips and thighs, £4,500.

BUM:

Buttock implants, £6,500;

Replacement buttock implants as one shifted and developed fluid, £4,000;

Liposuction to buttock, hips and thighs area for added smoothness, £3,500.

MEDICAL PROCEDURES I PERFORM MYSELF:

Fortnightly skin peels, monthly dermabrasion, monthly injectable fillers, botox bi-monthly, botox underarms yearly, botox to feet, six-monthly cosmetic tattooing, monthly teeth bleaching, £22,000 a year, or £220,000 for the last 10 years.

Hair extensions, £4,000 a year, or £72,000 for the last 18 years

And that comes to a grand total of £528,500, excluding hair! And Tony says that I am high maintenance – I cannot for the life of me imagine what he could possibly mean.

CHAPTER 19
Making An Honest Living

The tabloids like to say that I have spent more than £500,000 on plastic surgery, but you now know that is untrue, and that £500,000 is in fact the value of my surgery if I were to have paid for it. Had it not been for the deals I was able to do with some of the most trusted cosmetic surgeons in England, I would have had very little done.

Hollywood Looks was probably my best shot at make a million but it simply wasn't to be. Then I was scraping together a decent living working at home when Tony and I first set up house together and that went pear-shaped when I was branded a benefits cheat.

So how do I make a living as 'Real-Life Barbie'?

First of all, I run a free cosmetic surgery referral service. People contact me through my websites after seeing me on TV, or in newspaper and magazine articles and they want advice about plastic surgery, advice that I am happy to provide.

I am now in a position to refer them to surgeons all around the world, not just in England. I always find out what their objectives are, what they want to get out of the plastic surgery, and then I need to establish what size budget they have – sometimes, people have unrealistic targets and ambitions, and simply don't have enough money to achieve those objectives. I believe it is important to be honest with them and tell them that they will have to go away and save some more in order to have things done properly.

Where do they live? Are they prepared to travel?

You would not believe how many of these people want the same surgeons who have operated on me.

All of this takes a lot of my time, but it makes me feel good to know that I am pointing people in the right direction. If I appear on TV, it is not unusual to find hundreds upon hundreds of emails on my website the next day, and I always try to reply to everybody – apart from the cranks, of course.

I then contact the relevant surgeon and eventually I put the two parties together. If the procedure goes ahead as a result of the work that I have put in, the surgeon will then give me a percentage of whatever he makes from that consultation.

So as far as the would-be customers are concerned, they get a free service from me and the knowledge that the doctor I refer them to will be the best one for the job.

And then there is my media activity. I make many TV appearances, all over the world, and of course I get paid for it. On top of that, I get paid for the interviews I give to newspapers and magazines. It was tough during the recession, but I have never been afraid of hard work and will do whatever it takes to put food on the table, even if it has meant accepting less than I would have wanted for certain jobs I have done.

From time to time, I will do something for nothing if I believe that it might attract publicity which could, in turn, lead to other work. In many respects, it is a balancing act.

I find that I am doing increasing amounts of work for Japanese television – I think they are obsessed with women who have blonde hair and big tits, both of which I possess in abundance. The Japanese are very strange in as much as they are always making requests to film me doing stuff such as pushing a shopping trolley around Tesco or Sainsbury's. And then we end up talking about plastic surgery with the help of a translator.

I have also been the face of a private hospital in Cambridge for media purposes.

Then there is *OK!* Magazine, for whom Tony and I stage celebrity parties on a regular basis. It came about through attending a party at which we met Mark Moody, the social editor of OK! We started chatting and got on with each other right from the off. As a result, we were invited to further parties organised by *OK!*

It is a huge-selling magazine and the parties are attended by various celebrities, some of whom are A-listers, some of whom are not. The magazine takes lots of pictures and they appear in the next issue. It is as simple as that.

When I was developing HumanHi, I decided with Tony that we would throw a series of parties of our own, so I contacted Mark and asked if he could get *OK!* to come along and take pictures. "Sarah, as long as you can guarantee to me that there will be celebrities at your parties, then I can guarantee we will come along, take photos and put them in the magazine." You would be amazed how easy it is to get celebs to come along if they think they are going to get a free glass of bubbly and have their picture taken for *OK!* I found it hard to take in at first, but nothing surprises me any more.

And because our parties are featured in *OK!*, we have been able to get sponsorship, so we end up getting the venue for nothing, and we might also get free vodka, free energy drinks, free bottled water – it is all about product placement and making sure they are featured in the photo shoot.

It means that if, say, somebody has a clothes range that they want to advertise or promote, they will come to HumanHi and tell us that they want a party to launch their range. We quote a price, and in return we get *OK!* to send along a photographer and we arrange the venue and the free drink and suchlike. At the end of the day, everybody is happy. What we charge the clothes designer is a tiny fraction of what it might cost them to pay for the equivalent in advertising space, and they know that they are being featured in what is arguably the most popular magazine in Britain.

There are times when the parties can get out of hand, which is a danger when free alcohol is on the menu. On one occasion there was a woman at one of our parties who turned out to be a thoroughly nasty piece of work. It turned out that she was jealous of the fact that I'd had lots of plastic surgery, and she ended up trying to punch and kick me, as well as pinching me, just to see what my skin felt like. For reasons which we never did fathom, she also went for my PR. A quick phone call to the police soon sorted that one out.

I don't know why, but I do seem to attract what I consider to be more than my fair share of criticism and even hate mail.

While I get lots of emails on the website from people looking for help and wanting advice, there are also those who consider me to be some kind of evil freak. These people don't know my story, don't know I was a victim of domestic violence, so they assume that I must be a spoilt little rich girl who has spent all of my husband's hard-earned cash on my beauty treatments.

I have no problem with people criticising me, but I do wish that they would take the trouble to check out their facts before attacking me. The type of thing I receive usually follows these lines:

"You think you are so beautiful but you are not. You are really, really ugly, and you should be ashamed of yourself for spending your children's inheritance." Thank goodness for the delete button.

And then there is the other side of the coin, the people who tell me that

I am a breath of fresh air for telling it like it is. "You talk about plastic surgery in a way people can understand, and you are able to laugh at yourself. You are totally human in that respect and I think you are great." When I am feeling down, emails like that always bring a smile to my face and put a spring in my step. I especially love it when I get those sort of comments from women – that's when I feel that I am not wasting my time.

Next up are the men who want to marry me, even though I make no secret of the fact that I am happily married. What has particularly surprised me is the number of young men who contact me – maybe they see me as the mother they wish they had. Perish the thought!

When I get young lads telling me they want to do this, that and the other to me I usually answer them, letting them down as gently as I can. I think it's great, but Tony doesn't always see the funny side of a 20-year-old male lusting after his wife.

"They wouldn't want you if they knew what you were really like!"

"Thanks Tony."

"Listen to this one. He is only 19 and he wants me to sit on his face. Don't you think that's fantastic?"

"No, I do not Sarah. I think it is disgusting."

Then there are the lesbians who want to turn me. Funnily enough, none of them ever send picture of themselves, which I find a bit strange.

What may be the biggest surprise of all to you is to learn that lots of young girls contact me, saying they have stumbled across me on Facebook or wherever, and who they would love to have a mother like me.

"You are so open about plastic surgery, and when I grow up I am going to have it done to me too..."

And this raises a serious question, one that I often consider. Am I a good role model for young people? Let me answer that by first of all saying that I hope no young girl would ever repeat many of the mistakes that I made. But let's get something straight here – I am not encouraging young girls, or anybody else for that matter, to have plastic surgery. It is a choice for the individual to make, but if anybody asks for my advice, I will give it, regardless of age. Obviously, if I am giving an answer to a 12-year-old girl, it would be totally different to the response I would give to somebody or 22, 32, 42 or 52.

The sort of thing I hear is: "If when I get older and my looks don't improve and I end up looking like my mother then I would want to have something done to change my appearance. I want to have plastic surgery so that I can end up looking like you because I think you look amazing for your age."

I would reply to an email like that by thanking them for the compliments they had paid me and then go on to say that I was sure they wouldn't have to worry about plastic surgery, that they were probably stunningly beautiful girls who would make their own mothers proud. I would never, ever alienate a girl I had never met from her mother.

I tell them to listen to their mothers and say that if they want to contact me when they reach their twenties then I will be happy to help if I can.

Apart from anything else, as has been well enough documented in this book, I have had my own problems as a mother.

In fact, there was one story with Hannah that backfired spectacularly. I was approached by a magazine who wanted to do a piece on teenagers and botox, and was asked whether I would be interested in doing it with Hannah – when I told her there was £300 in it for her she said: "Sure, why not?"

I know what I am doing. Hannah first had botox in Spain when she was 15 years old. There was one main reason. Apart from the other things that it does, botox stops excess sweat from the forehead – Hannah dances professionally, so I was happy for her to have the injections if it would stop her sweating. Let's get something straight here – Hannah did not receive botox to remove wrinkles.

She is a well rounded girl, and I am very proud of her – in fact, she was so determined to disassociate herself from her father, that she had us change her surname to Burge at the first available opportunity.

I feel very strongly that if teenage girls are going to have botox then they should be allowed to have it injected by reputable practitioners, and so I thought this article could be a good thing. As far as I was concerned, it was going to be about teenage girls becoming so obsessed with their looks that they were considering using botox, and we could warn them about the dangers of going to some back-street quack who didn't know what they were doing.

A photographer turned up and said he wanted to take a picture of me giving Hannah an injection, so I had to explain to him that I didn't do that.

"But you do have needles in the house?"

"Yes, I do."

"Well in that case, I just need you to show me what would happen if you were to give her an injection then."

Before I knew what was happening, it was all over the tabloid press that I gave my daughter botox injections and along with the article was a photograph that supposedly proved it beyond all doubt – the photograph I had been stupid enough to pose for. And I was being branded as an irresponsible mother. As Hannah herself said later, would such a fuss have been made of this had the injections been administered under her arms?

Why do these things keep happening to me?

I have always tried to laugh at myself, no matter how serious the situation in which I find myself, so I called myself the 'Botox baddie', but by now the press were branding me 'Botox Barbie'. And there it was in black and white – I was giving my 15-year-old daughter botox injections. Anybody with half a brain would know it was a set-up, but, sadly, that is not how it worked out.

I was upset, but that was as nothing when compared with how Hannah felt when she saw the papers. She was mortified. Remember that this is a schoolgirl, somebody who then had to go and face her classmates. Needless to say, she went to school the day the article appeared and she took a right ribbing. I just thank God that she is tough enough to take it.

I don't know how she coped with it, but she did. I offered to go to the school but that was the last thing she wanted. As happens with these things, it began to die down, but then one of the newspapers decided to dredge it up all over again.

It was the only time in my life that I refused to do radio and TV interviews – they can do what they want to me, but not to my daughter. It was so unfair because, when all was said and done, I had done nothing wrong other than being a bit naive.

But get this – the offers started pouring in for Hannah, including $9,000 to appear in an American TV show. She turned it down because she did not want to be known for botox. I fully respect the right my children have to make their own decisions, but Hannah wants to attend a dance school, and the money she could have got from going to America would have helped enormously.

The worst part of the whole experience, however, was when I had a social worker knocking on my door because somebody had reported me as an unfit mother. Hannah had phoned me from school to tell me that she had been questioned by a social worker who had been accompanied by a plain clothes police officer, and they wanted to know all about the botox – she was only 15 at the time, and if I had been stupid enough to have given her injections then I would have been in serious trouble.

Hannah informed them that I had never given her botox, but the next thing I knew was that they were at the front door, wanting to ask me the same questions. Weeks had passed since the article originally appeared.

The conversation went something like this:

"Mrs Burge, it has been all over the newspapers that you give botox to your 15-year-old daughter. What do you have to say about that?"

"You have just spoken to my daughter – what did she tell you?"

"She said that you have never given her a botox injection."

"In that case, why have you come round to ask me the same question?"

The police officer then asked me what I said to my children before I went off to have cosmetic surgery. "That is none of your business, and it has nothing whatsoever to do with the reason for you coming to my home."

The line of questioning was offensive and entirely irrelevant. They even asked if my daughters saw me swathed in bandages. Call me old-fashioned, but it seems pretty obvious that if I go and have a facelift then I will come home with bandages on my face, but what on earth did that have to do with the allegations that I'd given Hannah botox injections?

"Why am I being victimised here? I have done nothing wrong. Nothing."

I later discovered that they were not bothered so much about what was going with Hannah as they were about Poppy, who was six years old at the time – did they honestly think that I would give botox to a six-year-old? No, but they did think that I had sat down and had a serious conversation with her about her having a boob job when she was older. An article had appeared in a woman's magazine and they had got hold of a copy of it and, yet again, had twisted things. Why oh why would I sit down with a six-year-old child and have a discussion with her about breast augmentation. She is six – she couldn't give a toss about breasts. All that she was interested in were her dolls and her computer games. Give me strength.

I suggested to the police officer that it might make more sense for the force to deal with the problem of teenagers taking drugs, stealing cars and having under-age sex instead of grilling me about a shot of botox that never happened. Eventually they told me that they accepted that my children were not at risk, but they did ask if I would in future keep them posted as to any potential stories that might appear in the media – and they were absolutely serious!

It turned out that the school had alerted the police. I was livid. How dare they allow my daughter to be interviewed by the police without first informing me. I had a heated telephone conversation with the teacher who had called in the authorities, who told me that she had every right to do so because she felt that Hannah was in danger. It was absurd. Tony grabbed the phone from me and informed her that he was going to get in touch with the press about the number of pupils who were taking cocaine. I don't think I have ever seen Tony so angry.

Thankfully, I have lots of good neighbours and friends who see these stories for what they are – if I was putting my children at risk, don't you think that those people would contact the authorities?

It was a horrible experience, one that taught me yet another lesson. I made up my mind that I would never again allow myself to be manipulated by the media. If there was going to be any manipulating to be done in future, then I was going to be the one who was pulling the strings, expect that it didn't turn out that way. As you will discover, I was to fall victim to the media again on more than one occasion. But I am a tougher person than some give me credit for, and I will keep bouncing back.

There is a serious note to all of this. Because I am so concerned that teenagers get the right sort of help and advice on cosmetic surgery, botox and fillers, I have set up a global campaign on my website www.thesarahburge.com, which is designed to point them in the right direction. Whether we like it or not, teenagers are obsessed with their looks and it is important that both they, and their parents, know the risks that they run by not properly checking out treatments and those who apply them.

CHAPTER 20
Conning The Conman

Throughout my life I have met many dubious characters, and I began to develop to a sixth sense about people. One such person was a man who passed himself off as Jonathan De Mornay, the brother of actress Rebecca De Mornay. We later discovered that his real name was Charles Lewis, but even that may not be true.

Tony was in Spain and had phoned me and as we spoke he started to tell me about this 'fabulously wealthy' man he had been introduced to who had been looking for investors for a deal involving cheap wine and vodka. He was guaranteeing that anybody who invested would treble their initial investment in no time at all. It all sounded too good to be true, and I wondered why somebody who was wealthy in his own right would ever need to involve investors.

But Tony seemed genuinely excited by it.

"What does he want from you Tony?"

"Nothing. He thinks that he probably has more than enough investors already."

I was due to join Tony a couple of days later in Marbella, where we have a place, and he told me that we would be having dinner with 'De Mornay' at one of the most exclusive hotels in the resort.

As we sat in the courtyard bar waiting for him, I looked up and saw this man swaggering towards us. I turned to Tony and said: "Is that him?"

"Yes Sarah, but keep your voice down. He is a very wealthy man."

"I tell you what he is Tony – he is a conman."

"Don't start. He hasn't even opened his mouth yet – how can you know?"

"I am telling you. I have been surrounded by people like him all my life. He is going to want something from you, I guarantee it."

De Mornay/Lewis didn't need to utter a word. I just knew.

"Hello, I'm Jonathan De Mornay, lovely to meet you."

I rose to shake his hand, told him it was lovely to meet him too and spent the night going through the motions.

I got the impression from the off that he realised I had seen straight through him because he went out of his way to pay me compliments, and to tell me that he had seen me on TV and had read all about me. He told me I looked fantastic – it was sickening. But hey, he was paying for a fabulous meal, as well as for the drink, so I decided just to go along with it and see where it took us.

When we sat down for dinner he kept getting up to go to the toilet, claiming he had bladder problems. Mmm...maybe, maybe not.

Tony was upset by my cynicism. "This man is very wealthy and very well connected, and we might be able to use his connections, so please keep your thoughts to yourself Sarah."

When De Mornay/Lewis was at the table he didn't stop talking. "I can count my true friends on the fingers of one hand," he said. "And Tony, you are one of them now."

I couldn't help myself. "You guys have only known each other for five minutes – how can you suddenly be best buddies?"

We had a daughter – he had a daughter. My parents had a dog – his parents had a dog. I had done TV work – he knew somebody who had worked on the same programme. He did and said everything he could think of to ingratiate himself into our lives.

The evening ended with him telling us to meet him at the hotel the next morning for breakfast, and he would bring his daughter, Katie, with him to meet Poppy. We agreed, and I could not believe how different two young girls could be. Poppy behaved like you would expect a typical young girl to behave, running around, having fun. Lewis's daughter – if indeed she really was – sat at the table and said next to nothing, speaking only when she was spoken to. It sent shivers down my spine.

Then there was his 'wife'. The very first time I met her, I just knew that something wasn't right – she was wearing glasses and she had thick frizzy hair, but my feeling was that the hair was definitely a wig and that she was hiding behind the glasses, almost as if it were all part of a disguise.

We spent a great deal of time with De Mornay/Lewis, and he was paying for everything, until eventually he announced that he was, after all, able to find room for Tony to invest in the wine and vodka deal – all that he needed was £10,000.

"You will get your money back in six weeks, three times over. Guaranteed."

I told Tony not to do it. It's the old adage – if it sounds too good to be true, it probably is. And it was. Tony was ready to hand over the money but I begged him not to. We came home to England, and I hoped that would be the last we would hear of De Mornay/Lewis, but then he asked if he could have a limousine delivered to our house. He was going to get his chauffeur to drive it to Spain but needed to leave it somewhere safe in the meantime.

Next, there was talk of De Mornay/Lewis coming back to London to celebrate his 50th birthday at the Dorchester, and he wanted us to come. Mysteriously, he never came back to London and the party did not happen.

Tony was still determined to invest. "Listen Sarah, what if I get somebody to go 50-50 with me, so that means I am only putting up £5,000, and he puts up the rest?" The plan was for Tony to ask Joe, a friend and colleague, to go in with him.

When Joe came round to the house and heard about the scheme he was really keen, but I told him: "Joe, if you hand over any money to this man you will never see it again. He is a conman. Period."

My husband was still convinced that I was wrong about this man, but Joe said: "Tony, you should listen to Sarah. I believe there is such a thing as women's intuition, and if she has a bad feeling about all of this, then maybe she is right. Listen to her."

But, of course, nobody did listen to me in the end, and Joe parted with his £5,000 and we parted with ours. Tony handed it over to De Mornay/Lewis, who repeated his assertion that we would receive £40,000 in six weeks.

Guess what? Six weeks went by and Tony contacted De Mornay/Lewis to be told the deal hadn't quite been done yet. Another six weeks went by, and then another six weeks, and all the while he kept telling us not to worry. "That's it. Our money has gone," I said.

The next excuse was that he had a passport problem and couldn't get to Switzerland to pick up the money. He then tried to blame the Spanish authorities for delaying things, and next he came up with some tosh about his wife wanting to divorce him.

We knew by now that the money had gone so we decided to string him along and kept persuading him to take us out to the finest restaurants, always making sure that he picked up the bill. We would go shopping and make sure that he was dragged along too and I would pick out designer clothes for Poppy and ask him to pay, telling him he could take it out of our profits. He could hardly say no, could he?

Poppy got a D&G dress out of it, Tony got a jacket and shoes, and I managed to get him to buy me some bits and pieces too. For a period of about six months, we took this man for as much as we could get out of him. It cost him a damn sight more than the money he had from us, and our only regret was that a friend of Tony's had ended up out of pocket.

There was one occasion when De Mornay/Lewis was wining and dining us at the exclusive and extremely expensive Las Dunas hotel in Marbella when I glanced over to the next table, and there was Hollywood actor Matt Damon and his family – it was the night before he was due to fly to London for the UK premier of The Bourne Ultimatum. It was a surreal experience. Poppy ended up playing with Damon's daughter, and the next thing we knew, we were talking to him. De Mornay/Lewis told Damon that his sister was the actress, Rebecca De Mornay, and Damon even told him that he could see the family likeness.

It all came to a head when he promised to take us on holiday to Sandy Lane in Barbados. It wouldn't have been so bad had he not involved Hannah and Poppy but he did, and they were both really excited, thinking that they were going on the holiday of a lifetime.

He had given us the dates and told us that he had booked our flights but we grew suspicious when there was no sign of any tickets, so we checked with the airline and it emerged that the tickets did not exist. He would have had us turn up at the airport with my two daughters and all our luggage and then find out that the whole thing was a wind-up. He didn't care that my two girls would have ended up in tears.

Tony phoned him to ask what was going on, and even then he wouldn't admit that there was no holiday, trying to convince my husband that he had booked and paid for first class tickets and they didn't always show up if you phoned up to check. He had no shame.

I grabbed the phone. "Jonathan, you disgust me. From the second I saw you I knew that you were a conman. I have lived and worked with them all my life. But the biggest mistake you made was to get my children involved and, for that, I am going to hunt you down like a dog."

I then decided to post a warning on my website because I didn't want other people to fall prey to this dreadful man. Among other things, he had promised to help me with an idea I'd had to launch an exclusive range of clothing, so I made up my mind to put together a press release announcing that 'billionaire [there is nothing to beat laying it on with a trowel] Jonathan De Mornay was going to help Sarah Burge with her clothing range launch...'

I then sat back and waited to see what would happen. Before long, the newspapers were contacting me, asking me who this man was, and I told them he was the brother of Rebecca, the actress. I just spouted the line he had given me. A couple of newspapers ran the story, as did a couple of magazines. Perfect.

Then, just as I had expected, I started to hear from people from all over the world who had also been conned by De Mornay/Lewis. They came from America, from Jersey, from Germany, from Switzerland, from Australia, and they were all saying the same thing – do not go near this man. All these people had fallen victim to him, handing over thousands of pounds that they never saw again.

We eventually got together with a group of his victims. The con was always slightly different, adapted to suit the individual, but it always involved relieving them of money for a scheme that couldn't possibly go wrong. They described a man with dark hair, but his hair had been blonde when we were dealing with him. And they described a beautiful wife, which simply confirmed my suspicions about the woman he had introduced to us as his wife – she had, indeed, been in disguise. Things like things only happened in the movies, surely?

The most upsetting case of all involved John Shelby, a man in his seventies, who ended up remortgaging his house. Having handed over several thousand pounds, De Mornay/Lewis told him that he needed more, and this poor man gave him more, and then some more, until eventually there was nothing left. Even his home had gone. This poor man ended up crying on my shoulder.

We went to the police in Huntingdon and the next thing we knew was that we were being contacted by a special team of investigators who offered us victim support and informed us that they were all too well aware of De Mornay/Lewis and his antics. There was even talk about a safe house.

I am glad to say that we have never heard from him again, although from time to time I still get emails and phone calls from people telling me about the latest scam they have heard about. Personally, I have no idea how people like De Mornay/Lewis can live with themselves. It is bad enough that they go around conning innocent people out of their hard-earned savings, but I wonder how they sleep at night or what goes through their minds when there is an unexpected knock at the door or a footstep behind them as they walk home in the dark.

Tony and I managed to get him to spend thousands on us and it makes me think that he did actually like us – he would never recover the sums of money he lavished upon us. For him, I think the con was just a job. He didn't see his victims as people, but as 'marks' or 'targets'.

There is actually a man out there called Jonathan De Mornay who is the genuine brother of Rebecca and, as far as I can ascertain, he is a wealthy man in his own right. I can only begin to guess how his reputation must have been sullied by the man who wormed his way into our lives.

CHAPTER 21
Into The Pink

I do not believe in standing still. You have to move on, and constantly reinvent yourself, and I have managed to do so through a medium that I have called Madame Pink. Everything I have done in my life has been achieved through drawing on my own life experiences, and it has been the same with this too.

Barbie and I have lots and lots in common – we are the same age, we both married our first love, plastic looms large in our lives (in her case it's what she is made of, in my case it is plastic surgery) and she was modelled on a German porn doll called Bild Lilli. Strange, but true.

So it got me thinking. If Barbie and I had all these things in common, how could I make something of the porn doll connection? I used to go whoring around London, so maybe I could reinvent myself yet again. And so I came up with Madame Pink.

I make no bones about it – I enjoy sex. Who doesn't? And I have made no secret of my passion for passion during television interviews because to deny it would be hypocritical.

But let me make it clear here and now that Madame Pink is a fantasy figure – a sexual fantasy figure who gets up to all sorts of mischief in a land of make believe. This is something else that has landed me in trouble because there are some people out there who cannot tell the difference between fact and fiction.

I get up in the morning and I make up stories which I then put on the Internet, and yes, I admit that to get into character I will sometimes dress up as, say, a nurse or a schoolgirl, but it is all done in the privacy of my own home when my children are at school. And it is all perfectly innocent. Tony is often the beneficiary because it goes without saying that if I am making up a sexual fantasy there are times when I either get very turned on or when I want to act it out with the man in my life. I can assure you that I have never heard him complain.

And so the two of us role-play, but if I decide to put the story or fantasy on my website, I always try to inject a bit of humour. I suppose you would describe it as Carry On With Bells On. Yes, there is always a basis in fact, but these are not real stories and sometimes I amaze even myself with some of the filth that pours out of my mouth.

I have a website, www.madamepink.co.uk and there are people out there who are convinced that it is a front for a knocking shop, and that I am some kind of prostitute. Personally, I find it all a little bit sad that there are so many individuals out there who apparently have no sense of humour, and who take everything so bloody seriously.

These stories may eventually find their way into top-shelf magazines or a series of books, but it will all be done tongue in cheek.

Sure enough, however, one of the tabloids portrayed me as a £500-per-hour prostitute – they had taken some of the stuff on the website as gospel and, of course, did not bother to check their facts. I had written: "For 500 smackers an hour, I can be whatever my master wants me to be." But it wasn't real. I had written the piece through the eyes of a blow-up doll, not a real person, and certainly not me!

I got in touch with the paper and informed them that if I was charging for sex I would be putting another nought on the end of the figure they had come up with. They refused to publish a retraction but in the end it probably didn't do me any real harm because it attracted lots of publicity for the website and the people who checked out the site as a result would have been deeply, deeply disappointed if they thought that they were going to be able to hire me for sex at any price because it just wouldn't happen.

The blow-up doll story was based on a real-life experience I'd had during my time with Jock when there was this man who paid him on the understanding that I would just lie there and say nothing, and show no emotion or feeling. Whatever turns you on.

I enjoy being Madame Pink, although I know how strange it must seem. How many mothers get their children ready for school and then, once they have gone, sit down to compose a filthy yarn? With apologies to the likes of Ted Hughes, John Betjeman and Andrew Motion, I would describe myself as the Poet Laureate of Filth.

I have a case full of props and costumes, and there are days when I prance around dressed like a porn star, brandishing a whip, because if I dress in character then I find it much easier to get my inspiration. In saying that, there are days when I can just throw on a jogging suit and get into character – it depends upon my frame of mind when I get up in the morning.

We have also done some slapstick videos with my filmmaker friend Martin Marshall. Yes, I wear low-cut blouses and short skirts but we do these things because they are funny and sometimes we can't film for laughing. If you conjure up images of Benny Hill of the Confessions series then you will not be too far off the mark. It is good clean fun. Sorry, let me rephrase that – it is good filthy fun. Sex should be fun after all.

There is one video where I pretend to be a naughty schoolgirl, another where I am a nurse. We do them unscripted and when Martin puts the finished product together he speeds them up, again a bit like Benny Hill. We also did one where I pretended to go and see a psychiatrist because

I supposedly needed help for my sex addiction and, of course, the idea is that I try to seduce the psychiatrist.

Occasionally we do outdoor shoots too, and those have been hysterical because the sort of places we would want to film usually attract people, so we always need to have a coat handy, and we always need to be ready to leg it. He has filmed me on the beach, in a farmer's field and he even once filmed me sprawled over the altar in a church, wetting myself in case anybody came in.

Perhaps the strangest of all was the shoot we did at Martin's local gymnasium. He actually contacted them first and told them what we wanted to do – the idea was that I was a scantily-clad schoolgirl and I was to work myself into a state of arousal while working out on the various pieces of apparatus. It really was harmless fun, where all I was doing was making panting noises and suchlike as he filmed me lifting weights, but you can imagine the looks we got from our fellow gym users.

I sat down afterwards and imagined some of these people going home to their wives. "Darling, you are not going to believe me when I tell you what happened at the gym today..."

Most people go to work in an office...

CHAPTER 22
Heavy Metal

When Tony was involved in the aluminium business, he got a phone call one day from a guy who told him that he needed some specialist equipment for a night club, but he was reluctant to go into too much detail over the phone. He was based in Biggleswade, so Tony agreed to go and see him.

His name was Mark. We christened him Pervy Mark and he looked like Ian Drury, the singer, right down to the gammy leg.

I tagged along with Tony because we were planning to go out for lunch after his meeting, Eventually we found this place and it was like walking into a black hole – everything was black, and I mean everything. To be honest, it was pretty creepy.

Next door was a sex shop, which was attached to the club. When we met Mark he got straight down to business, telling Tony he needed a cross, a cage and a chair on which men sit while their female partner urinates all over them – it is called a 'Pissy chair'. Somehow, Tony managed to keep his face straight as Mark delivered his wish list, but then he realised that this was an opportunity to make some serious money.

All this equipment would have to be custom-made. A bespoke 'Pissy chair' - have you ever heard anything like it in all your life?

These things needed to be made to a certain specification because, believe it or believe it not, there were health and safety issues involved. Mark needed to know that if, for example, a 20-stone man was strapped into the 'Pissy chair', it would take his weight.

After Tony had taken the order and satisfied himself that he could get the stuff built, Mark said: "The two of you will have to come along to one of our party nights. I reckon you would really enjoy yourselves. Besides, you need to see what your gear is going to be used for."

It transpired that this was a proper family business – Mark's wife was a dominatrix, who charged God-knows-what to men who were prepared to lie back and think of England, or whatever, while she whipped them.

We duly accepted the invitation, along with the instruction that we had to turn up dressed all in black. The evening started with a meal in Huntingdon and at first we weren't all that keen on going, but after a few drinks we decided that it might be a bit of fun, so off we went.

Because we'd had several drinks, we had to leave our car and get a taxi home to get changed into black clothes, and then we had to get another taxi to Biggleswade. It was like walking into the Seventh Circle of Hell. The place was heaving, and there was somebody attached to a cross with somebody else whipping him, there were men in nappies, there were men wearing dog chains, and there were women walking around kicking the men.

So this is what a fetish party was like. Most people, I believe, have an image in their mind of the people who go to fetish and sex parties – they probably see most of them as big, fat men and women. Well I am here to tell you that that is not the case at all. I was well and truly flabbergasted.

Everywhere I looked there were stunning women and fit young men. Tony wandered off and I began to get a bit worried about him being seduced by a young woman.

I caught sight of Tony. "All right mate?"

"Sorry, do I know you?" asked Tony.

"Yeah, you were in here the other day talking to Mark about having some gear built for him. I am Gary."

And then the penny dropped with Tony. While we had been in the club there had been a builder who had been doing some work for Mark and had come over to say hello. In Tony's defence, it was hardly surprising that he didn't recognise Gary because this big, butch builder was standing there having a conversation with my husband while wearing nothing more than a nappy and holding a dummy in his right hand And he wasn't in the slightest bit self-conscious about it either.

I decided that I needed a drink, but there is a golden rule among fetishists, and that is that you don't get drunk because when whips and suchlike are concerned it can get dangerous. I was staggering from room to room with Mark hanging on to me.

Our evening ended with me being asked by this little man who reminded me of Jock to tie him to the cross and whip him. I discovered that I enjoyed it and the harder I hit this bloke, the more he seemed to enjoy it. I then realised that not only was Tony watching me, but so was just about every other person in the club – the poor man's body was covered in stripes where I had struck him with the whip, but he had loved every single second of it.

The only thing was that I had overdone it and the bloke ended up in a lot of pain, but he had asked me to do it to him. The next day, Mark called Tony and told him that in all the time he had been running fetish parties he had never once had a complaint, but more than 50 people had complained to him about my behaviour. Whoops!

"If you bring your wife again, you will have to keep her under control Tony," he said. Thankfully, I did not do any permanent damage, although how on earth he explained it to his wife when he got home I will never know – he had told me he was married but that his wife didn't know what he got up to.

And that was my first experience of a fetish party. One never to be forgotten, or repeated.

Tony realised there was a market for all this kit, so he had it made in flat-pack format in order that it could be used by couples in the privacy of their own homes and could then be taken apart and hidden underneath the bed so that Granny wouldn't see it when she came for the weekend.

Sadly, Mark's club went bust, but Tony is still able to supply crosses and suchlike to order.

CHAPTER 23
Carry On Doctor

As I have made clear, I was always happy to refer people to plastic surgeons who had worked on me, and one such surgeon was a doctor I will call Bhuto Balan, who had performed a facelift and breast reduction on me, and had done an excellent job. He was based at a hospital in London at the time.

I guess that I was sending him around 15 patients a week, and although he carried out consultations all over the country, most of the surgery he performed happened at the London hospital.

He turned round at one point and said that most of the patients were coming from other parts of the country, and he didn't think that I should get paid anything for them. I was flabbergasted. Whether a patient came from London, from Manchester or from Timbuktu, surely if I was the person who was arranging the introductions, then I was entitled to payment?

But he didn't see it that way, so we ended up falling out. If he had told me that he thought the commission I was charging him had been too high then I might have been prepared to renegotiate it, but he didn't. He just stopped paying me.

Meanwhile, I struck up a friendship with Dr Balan's secretary, who had a son that was the same age as Hannah, and they also hit it off. Let's call her Helen, and she ended up coming round to our house fairly regularly.

I will never forget her first visit to our home. She must have downed three bottles of wine, and ended up making me look normal. To be frank, her behaviour was outrageous, but she stopped Tony and I in her tracks when she claimed that surgery was being performed in return for sex at the hospital. She was alleging that if, for instance, a woman wanted a breast enlargement but couldn't afford it, if she agreed to have sex with the doctor, in return he would perform the procedure, but at a hugely reduced rate.

She claimed that the sex took place in a nearby hotel. Helen then looked outside and realised we had a spa in the garden. Without further ado, she stripped off her clothes, ran into the garden and jumped in. Her son, remember, was upstairs with our daughter. And Tony's children were also staying with us for the weekend.

Tony then took his clothes off, looked at me and said: "Come on Sarah, we may as well go and join her."

We joined her, but she was totally out of control, playing with herself and trying to grab Tony's privates as well. I am very open and liberal when it comes to sex, but this had come as a complete shock to me, especially coming on top of what she had alleged about the doctors.

Eventually, we all came back inside and Tony took his kids home. As the night wore on she was continuing to drink, but I was still speechless when she made a pass at me. Before I knew what was happening, she was on top of me, and she was snogging me and groping me, telling me how much she loved me. I didn't want to know, but this woman wasn't taking no for an answer.

Tony found it funny at first, but soon realised that this was no laughing matter when I told him that if didn't get her off me then I was going to have to hit her. Thankfully, before Tony could do or say anything, she passed out. Finally, the drink had taken its toll – it was like a scene from a bad film. We managed to put her to bed and let her sleep it off.

The next morning she was nursing the hangover from hell and pretended to remember nothing of the previous afternoon and evening, asking if she had acted like a complete idiot.

I never did say anything to anybody about Helen's allegations, but there is not the slightest doubt in my mind that she was telling us the truth.

CHAPTER 24
Oh Brother

On January 13, 2010, I received the following email:

Dear Sarah,

I am a TV Producer from Big Brother and I am currently casting the final set of housemates for the series that starts in the summer.

I wondered if you have ever thought about auditioning for the show? If you have I would like to offer you a fast track audition in London on 5th Feb. It is a day's audition for selected people only. If this is something you might be interested in, please let me know.

Kind Regards,

Naomi Channell

Assistant Producer, Big Brother 11

I have never been a fan of *Big Brother* – in fact it was the one reality TV show I had always said I would never do. I would love to do *I'm A Celebrity! Get Me Out Of Here!* This may come as a surprise, but I would have no fears or qualms about the bushtucker trials, or about eating bugs and having rats run all over my body. I have had more than my fair share of rats running over my body during my lifetime.

But I knew that this was going to be the final series of *Big Brother* and that Channel 4 would want to go out with a bang. And there was also the small matter of a first prize of £100,000 plus all that time on television to let the public know what I was all about, so I thought: "Why not?" I wasn't too thrilled about the prospect of being away from my family for weeks on end, but hey, I could always walk out – and that would get me even more publicity. So I got back to Naomi and told her that I was interested. They came back to me immediately, told me they were delighted, and confirmed that I would be taking part in a fast-track audition, which meant that I would not have to queue up with hundreds of other hopefuls.

Everything was done by email. There were no phone calls. At this point I contacted my agent and asked him to speak to Endemol on my behalf, just to try and get a feel for the lie of the land really, but they refused to talk to him and said they would only deal with me. Within days, I had been given a date for my audition.

I knew that I needed an outfit, so I asked Charlotte to help me because she is the most creative person I know. As we were talking, everything came flooding back and I apologised again for everything that I had put her through all those years earlier.

"Mum, it doesn't matter now. You did what you had to do, what you thought was right. I didn't understand it at the time, but now I do. You had to fight for your right to get out of that relationship and I am fine with it," she said. And I genuinely believe that she has been able to put it all behind her. But it eats away at me all the time.

Incredibly, she has turned out to be one of the most balanced individuals I know, and she doesn't have a malicious bone in her body. She is a lovely girl, who now lives with her father.

The day before the audition, I had appeared on the *Alan Titchmarsh Show*, during which Nick Ferrari, the TV and radio journalist, announced that he thought it obscene that I had spent so much on plastic surgery, accused me of spending my children's inheritance and then launched into an attack on my mothering skills – quite an achievement for a man who had never been in my home and had never spoken to any of my daughters or, indeed, to any member of my family.

I patted his hand and said: "Don't worry about it Nick because it costs me more to fuel up my yacht."

"You have a yacht?"

"Well not any longer Nick, because the recession hit us too, so we had to sell it to pay for some plastic surgery I wanted." There are times when I just love being me, and winding up pompous journalists is one of those times.

The *Big Brother* audition was being held in Wembley at 9am so I booked myself into a nearby hotel to make sure that there were no dramas about getting there on time, and I wore bright pink high-heeled shoes, jeans and a bright pink, off the shoulder top that can also be worn as a dress.

I walked into Wembley Arena and there were signs everywhere. I thought it would take 15 minutes or so, but I ended up being there all day – and it seemed that half of that time was spent following these signs and trying to find where I was meant to go.

The first room I entered contained about 100 people. Fast-track audition? No queueing up? Who were they kidding? I was asked for my name and number – at this stage I had been given the number 10,092. And then I had to have my picture taken.

Next, I was handed a form and was told to fill it in. I looked around to see if I recognised anybody, but no. I decided to phone Tony and tell him to come and get me. This was not what I had been promised.

I would do *Celebrity Big Brother* if they asked nicely, but there was no way that I was going to go through a marathon audition process, especially since they had approached me in the first place. Tony told me not to be so stupid, and to just get on with it and see what happened.

"They will probably get rid of you anyway Sarah," he said. "You will drive them mad." Somebody saw me on the mobile phone and told me to put it away, so now I was stuck. I decided that Tony was right and that I should give it my best shot and see what happened.

After I filled in the form I was told to stand in another line and wait. We were told not to talk to anybody else, unless we had been given permission to do so. This was like being back at school.

I was then shown into a room where I was told that I had three minutes to tell a group of judges about myself. I started off by telling them I had been a convent schoolgirl who had fallen by the wayside, and I knew that I had their attention. I managed to drop in a mention of being chosen as the Virgin Mary and having sex for money next to Victoria Station when I was still a schoolgirl. I still had their attention. And I managed to squeeze in the fact that I'd had sex with a Hollywood actor, worked for a villain and been beaten to a pulp. I could see it in their faces. They were thinking: 'Is this woman for real?' But I also knew that they loved me.

I had to wait a few minutes and then was told that I had passed that stage and would be moving on to the next part of the audition process. Wasn't I delighted? Wasn't I proud of myself? No I wasn't. I just wanted to get the thing over and done with.

"You will be going up stairs to fill in another form. Make sure you get some water because this could easily take you four hours," I was told. I have never seen anything like it. A form? It was more like a book, and they wanted every detail of my life. Obviously, nobody had time to read that before they moved us on to the next part of the audition – I don't mind admitting that I was mentally shattered by now. So much for the quick in and out audition I had been hoping for.

And on we went, this time into a room with two judges and 11 other

Big Brother wannabes.

We were asked if we would rather be rich or famous, and I decided to take control by announcing that I was both. One of the judges asked the group: "What do you think she is famous for?"

Eventually, a girl said: "You don't look like you are rich."

"And you don't look like you come from Peckham," I replied. I was fairly sure that I was getting Brownie points for taking control. Nobody, of course, managed to guess why I was famous.

The woman next to me then butted in and said: "Oh my God, if you put somebody like her into the house, the rest of us have no chance." With that, I was ushered out of the room and told I had passed through another level. They took me through Wembley Arena, through the Big Brother eye and sat me down on a stool, where they left me for a while.

And then came the voice. "This is *Big Brother*. We don't like glamour girls in *Big Brother*, so why are you auditioning?"

"Well, for a start, you asked me to audition, and second of all, thank you so much for the compliment but the truth is that I am far too old to be a glamour girl."

"You didn't put your age on your form – who old are you?"

"I am 49, and I have blown half a million quid on plastic surgery..."

I was in there for ages, and started to wonder if I would ever get out.

I was asked how I would inter-act with the other housemates. "I will be their Yummy Mummy. I will tuck them up in bed at night and tell them filthy stories," I replied. "And that's all folks!"

"Thank you very much. *Big Brother* will let you know."

I eventually emerged from Wembley Arena at 6pm, and I was done in. Tony was waiting for me, and we set off home with me convinced that I would never hear from them again.

During my audition I was asked thousands of questions, but one that sticks in my mind was: "What do you like about *Big Brother*?"

My reply? "Absolutely nothing, other than the fact that Endemol [the production company that makes the programme] has stumbled upon something that speaks volumes about today's society. It's a bit like voyeurism, and I am into all that sort of stuff." I have never watched it and I don't like it – for me, it's like watching paint dry.

But £100,000 is an awful lot of money, and I couldn't very well turn up my nose at the opportunity to further my career without having to pay for it, could I? No, of course I couldn't.

If I did get in, I had some concerns. For instance, I hoped that I would not have to cook for the other housemates. I can just about manage spaghetti bolognaise, I can open a can and I can manage anything that goes in a microwave, but other than that, I am absolutely hopeless, as my two ex-husbands, three daughters, numerous former lovers and current husband will all confirm. Stick a recipe book in my hand and I will find a way of cocking it up. Maybe it's because I don't have a huge attention span, so I tend to lose interest – I always want to be moving on to the next thing.

If I have to cook for more than one other person apart from myself, I will screw it up. Guaranteed. There have been times when Tony has been away on business, and I have announced that I will make dinner – everybody either runs for the hills, or makes their excuses and leaves!

There was a casserole dish that I made for the family – a real achievement as far as I was concerned. Nobody would eat more than one mouthful of it, but the worst thing of all was that when I put it into the dog's bowl, even he turned up his nose and refused to eat it. That was when I realised that I wasn't meant to be within a million miles of a kitchen. I blew up a microwave on another occasion by putting a can in it. That was not a pretty sight.

When we invite people round for a meal they always ask: "You are not cooking are you Sarah?"

So if Endemol wanted to screen a mass murder, putting me in charge of the kitchen would have been the way to achieve it.

Three weeks had passed since my Wembley audition when they contacted me to tell me that I was through to the next stage – another bloody audition! I had to meet somebody outside BB's Muffins in Hammersmith before being taken off for another series of interviews and tests.

My contact would be carrying a red umbrella and I had to walk up to her and give her the password. 'Harold'. As it happens, there is more than one branch of BB's Muffins in Hammersmith, and I, of course, went to the wrong one. It was chucking down with rain, so there were lots of people walking by carrying red umbrellas, but it was pretty obvious that none of them had anything at all to do with *Big Brother*. And guess who didn't have an umbrella with them? So I was getting soaked.

I had a number to ring in case of emergency and after a while I called it. "I am meant to be with you, but I am not. Where are you?"

"We are outside BB's Muffins."

"You can't be, because I am standing outside BB's Muffins, and I can't see you."

"Well you are obviously standing outside the wrong BB's Muffins. We will wait for you, but this is not very good, is it?"

She gave me directions, and all that I wanted to do was to tell her what she could do with her audition, but I bit my tongue and set off in search of the next branch of BB's Muffins. Eventually I found it but I couldn't see anybody with a red umbrella so I went inside to have a look around – still nothing. By now I was thoroughly pissed off and as I walked out I saw somebody standing by the door swinging the tiniest of red umbrellas

– she didn't even have the thing open! It was the woman from *Big Brother*, and it was clear that she knew I was looking for her.

"At last," I said. "Thank God I've found you."

"Password."

"Harold. But before you say another word, I am desperate for the toilet."

She pointed me in the direction of the public toilets and when I got there I realised it was one of those turnstile affairs where you have to pay to get in, but I had no change and decided to try and climb over it. I got stuck, and not only did I get stuck, but my trousers split. In the end, a guy on his way out of the gents helped me over but I dropped my bag and the contents spilled all over the floor. So I am standing there, dripping wet through, trousers split, contents of my bag on the floor, wondering what on earth I was doing there.

And when I looked at myself in the mirror I wanted to scream – I looked bloody awful. But I staggered back to the woman with the red umbrella, who led us to a big old Victorian building they had hired for the day.

I was shown into a room along with another 12-16 people, a couple more producers and a big mirror on the wall. They told us that we should give ourselves a round of applause for getting so far. Most of the others did, but I couldn't see the point.

We all had to bring something with us that we felt summed up who we were. The first girl to get up had brought a Bible with her and droned on about how good a person she was. Give me strength. A gay man stood up and announced that he had brought a cake with him because he enjoyed baking. "Well at least we won't starve," I said. "It means you won't have to taste my cooking."

And so it went on. I was last, and I had brought a syringe with me. "I have brought this because I go around injecting botox into 15-year-olds," I announced. You will remember I told you the story about Hannah and the supposed botox injections – well, it had been in the news at around about this time, so I decided to make a meal of it. Almost in unison, the group said: "I know who you are..."

"Right, that's enough number 92, sit back down," I was told. I wanted to say: "I am not a number. I am a human being," but I thought better of it.

We were then asked to imagine that we were in the house – of the group who had just had their say, who would we vote out. Without any hesitation at all, one of the men pointed at me and said: "Her. She is totally plastic and does not live in the real world."

I had almost certainly lived more in the real world than the rest of these people put together. "Blimey, don't hold anything back baby," I said to him. What really hurt was that several other people decided to support him and agreed that they would vote me out too. Didn't any of these people realise that I was having a laugh. By now I was beginning to wonder if it was worth all the trouble – was this what it was going to be like if I got into the house?

At this point the producers said that they were going to leave us for 15 minutes, during which they wanted us to have a discussion as to why we thought that we had been colour-coded. I hadn't noticed, but all our numbers were different colours. And I then realised that myself and the guy who was the first to say he would vote me out were wearing the same colour, so I went over and sat beside him. We actually came to the conclusion that there was no rhyme nor reason to it, and that they would be having great fun filming us all coming up with our various theories.

After a few moments, I was aware that one of the men was looking closely at me, inspecting me. "How much plastic surgery have you had?"

he asked me, and before I knew it, the entire conversation was about cosmetic surgery. I didn't know whether this was a good thing or a bad thing, but I did realise that I had once again managed to upstage everybody else in the room without even trying.

Half an hour later, the producers entered the room and announced how pleased they were that we had all been getting on so well, and then they gave each of us a sticker bearing words such as 'Bimbo', 'Drama Queen', and 'Wannabe'. We had to put our stickers on the people we thought best fitted the description. Guess what? They put every bloody sticker onto me.

"Okay, thank you very much everybody. We will let you know..."

I couldn't make up my mind whether being singled out had been a good thing or a bad thing, but I reassured myself with the knowledge that at least it meant the rest of the group had noticed me, and surely that was what this dreadful programme was all about?

They contacted me later that day to tell me that I had made it through to the final selection process. Not another audition?

"We need you up at Shepherd's Bush on Monday morning at 9am for a psychiatric evaluation," I was told. Psychiatric evaluation? Oh dear!

I agreed to go along, and felt pretty relaxed about it all when the shrink told me that whatever I said to him would be treated in confidence. Yes, he had to write a report on me, but no, he would not be revealing any of what I might tell him.

He started off my saying: "Right then Sarah, tell me about your life..."

I was supposed to be with him for an hour, but four-and-a-half hours later I was still sitting with him. He was gobsmacked, and he said something that resonated with me. "You know Sarah," he said. "Everybody thinks that you are the fake, but you are not – you are very, very real. I can't tell you everything I am going to put in my report on you, but I can tell you that I am going to recommend that they include you in the show because you are a tabloid's wet dream. Nobody could make up your story."

In the afternoon I had to speak to a psychologist, and it seemed to me that he was determined to dissect everything that I said to him. When I told him about an experience, he wanted to know how I felt when it was happening to me. This was heavy stuff, but I got the feeling that this man could not make me out, and he was clearly shocked when I told him that I had refused to press charges against Faisal all those years earlier.

So that brought another day in the process to an end. Would this ever be over? Maybe, but not quite yet. Next I was told that they wanted to do a telephone interview. "We will call you at 4pm on Friday, when we will be asking you lots more questions about your life," I was told. I was getting pretty fed up with all of this, but agreed to go along with it and, sure enough, the phone rang at 4pm on the dot and I was subjected to a pretty painless telephone interview. They already knew most of what I told them anyway.

But then they wanted to speak to me over the phone again on the Tuesday of the following week. Perhaps they were seeing how far they could push me before I finally snapped, before I lost my patience with the entire process. I had come this far, and I had made up my mind that I was going to see it through to the bitter end, regardless of the outcome.

They wouldn't let go of the Madame Pink part of my life, wanting to know precisely what it involved and how much money I made through it. In the end, I decided to tell them what I thought they wanted to hear.

Back and forth it went. "You haven't quite made it yet, Sarah, but you are through to the next stage. We are now in the process of drawing up our final shortlist, and we will be back in touch soon to let you know."

To be fair to them, Endemol do extensive checks on everybody who goes into the *Big Brother* house, and they are to be applauded for that. They want to make sure that there are no issues with depression, that there is no dependency upon prescription drugs, that there are no suicidal tendencies. Yes, they are desperate for couples to have sex on live reality television, but they do not want anybody to kill themselves in front of the nation.

Still it wasn't over. I was asked to do an audition tape, giving my reasons for wanting to be in *Big Brother*, so I climbed into the spa, Tony switched on the camcorder and off I went, glass of champagne in hand. "Once upon a time there was a posh little convent schoolgirl who was always in the confession box, confessing her sins to the Father. She loved everything pink and silky but she didn't like dolls, preferring instead to swing around poles. And 40 years later she has laid herself bare for the *Big Brother* auditions, to scream, 'Please let me sin'." I waffled on and summed it up by saying: "I am going to inject a breath of fresh air into British television. Oh yes, and I forgot to tell you – I will be so good in *Big Brother*."

It was sheer hard work but, finally, I was sent a contract that confirmed I had made the final shortlist. It guaranteed me the princely sum of £1 plus expenses. I signed it and sent it off, but then they wanted two references, one of which had to come from Tony. I then tried to return to normal life until the big day arrived.

I had been sworn to secrecy, and I hadn't even told my children. The only person who knew was Tony. It had been made abundantly clear to me that if it leaked out that I might be appearing in *Big Brother* then I would be heading down the road.

So you can imagine my horror when, one Sunday in June, the phone started ringing off the hook with people wanting to know all about *Big Brother*. People I didn't know started contacting me through Facebook, asking for the lowdown. I hadn't the foggiest idea what was going on.

It was all over the News Of The World, and I was in a blind panic. I was under contract not to say anything, yet the News Of The World knew. There were photographers outside our house. I remember the date for a very good reason – it was 6 June, my Dad's birthday, and we had planned to go out and help him celebrate. No chance.

I was told not to leave my house. And I then had to sit down with Hannah and explain what was going on – I had actually written her a letter and the idea was that she was to open it after I had gone, but now I had to come clean. She thought it was great, especially when all her friends phoned and told her that they thought it was great that her Mum was going into *Big Brother*.

And then it clicked. It was the producers who had tipped of the newspapers so that they could build up the interest before the programme started. I could understand why they had done it, but I was really pissed off they hadn't taken me into their confidence. It was my Dad's birthday, and they had no right to ruin it. Quite apart from that, it was also the anniversary of Trevor's death, so this was an important day in the lives of my entire family.

In the end, I went into the back garden and dived over the back fence while Tony and Poppy got into the car and apparently drove off – when he was convinced that nobody had followed them, Tony brought the car round the back, I jumped in and off we went to see my parents. The day was further ruined by the fact that my phone kept ringing while we were out having Dad's birthday meal.

The following day I had to go to the station at Huntingdon. I was told to come on my own, which meant tearful farewells to Poppy and Tony. Poppy had given me Honey, her toy bunny rabbit, Tony had given me a kiss. It felt like I was heading off to start a prison sentence, although even in jail you are allowed to make phone calls, but I knew that I couldn't.

And off I went to Elstree, via King's Cross, where I was met by one of the team and asked to give the secret password. "Harold." I soon became pretty sick and tired of that name because it seemed to feature at the start of just about every single conversation that I had with employees of Endemol, who make *Big Brother*. I began to wonder what would happen if, when I was asked for the secret password, I replied: "Hilda." But I decided not to find out.

I asked myself time and time again why I was putting myself through this. It would have been totally different had I applied to go on the show, had I really wanted to appear on it, but I didn't. I had just somehow allowed myself to be swept along.

I had been instructed to dress to the nines, and was happy to do so, although on that first train I could feel the eyes of dozens of businessmen boring into me. I was wearing a short (very short) skin-tight skirt and a blouse slashed down the front and secured only by a brooch – otherwise I would have been showing off my tits to everybody on the train. So yes, maybe I would understand why there were so many eyes on me.

With me I had a case that was packed to overflowing – well I had to take enough clothes to cover for the possibility that I might be going into the *Big Brother* house for three months. I had packed some pretty unusual outfits - schoolgirl, nurse, Bunny Girl, air steward, kinky mistress, Miss Whiplash. I was determined that if I was going to be giving up my life for all these weeks then my housemates and the rest of the nation were going to find out what I was all about.

The case was heavy but, thankfully, when I got to King's Cross, somebody offered to carry it for me.

Other contestants were starting to arrive, but I quickly realised that none of them were smartly dressed. Why had they made such a point of asking me to look the part then? I was taken to a hotel, where I was relieved of my personal possessions, including money, writing material and my phone. The game had begun.

I was introduced to six other people and we were told that we would be the Yellow Team. Oh, and I was no longer Sarah. I was LT082. The group I was with included a former model, a singer and a former Miss England. We were a motley crew, but I couldn't help wondering why we had all been put together. Nothing happens by chance with TV. Nothing.

That first day was a full one, during which we were subjected to interviews on camera and photo shoots. We were also asked some very stupid questions, and I responded by giving them very stupid answers. I was asked how I how feel if I didn't get into the show and I replied: "If I don't get in, it will be one of television's biggest disasters."

We were sent to bed and told to be up bright and early the next day, and by 7am I was all made up and ready for action. It was easy enough for me because I have to get up every day to get the kids to school, but some of the others seemed to find it a challenge. I was the oldest member of our group so decided to assume the role of mother, making them tea and then getting into a routine of telling them stories each day and tucking them into bed at night.

We were told that we were all going to be meeting the press, but that we would have just one minute with each journalist. What sort of serious conversation can you have in 60 seconds? So I decided to have some fun instead.

At this stage, there were 80 would-be contestants and we were put into four rows, each comprising 20 people. A whistle was blown and the people in the front row spoke to an assigned journalist for one minute. Then the whistle blew and the second row stepped forward, and so on.

When it came to my turn I was asked: "Why do you want to be in *Big*

Brother?"

"So that I can show you my tits," was my considered reply. I went on to say that I felt that I could educate and shock viewers at the same time, while sparking controversy with the entire nation.

It seemed to do the trick because the next thing I knew was that I was being asked if I would show my tits in *Heat* magazine. "Absolutely delighted to do so," I said. "Just as long as the price is right, of course. These 32GGs are natural assets you know.

The day flew by, and I have to admit that I enjoyed it, especially when we had to do another bit of filming and they asked each person to come up with a catchphrase that they felt best summed them up. Mine was: 'I used to be such a nice girl'.

And then it was Wednesday, 9 June, the launch day. And still I hadn't a clue whether or not I was going to be in the house.

I was up at 4am, hair washed and make-up applied. I was raring to go, ready to do battle. We were at the studios by 7am and, upon arrival, we were given breakfast.

Then we decided to have some fun at *Big Brother*'s expense. The girls in my group asked if I would help them with their false eyelashes and I readily agreed to do so. I had a feeling that there would probably be hidden cameras so I then produced a syringe that I had hidden away and pretended to inject botox filler into everybody – just as I did so, members of the production team walked in and asked what the hell I thought I was doing. I explained that I was just making everybody look their best. "You can't do that," I was told in no uncertain fashion.

Then came rehearsal time. I wanted to look different and stand out from the crowd, so I wore a silver dress and headpiece and kept Honey the rabbit with me at all times. We were all ushered to the *Big Brother* set and I don't mind telling you that it was like being a piece of meat in a cattle market. What a bloody circus.

Each of us was given a number and a place to stand. I was now No33.

At 4.30pm a list of housemates was released to the press and I wasn't on it. Tony knew, but I didn't, of course. If I had known that I was being put through this pantomime for nothing, they wouldn't have seen me for dust. The producers had said, however, that an extra person whose name wasn't on the list would be included, so Tony had his fingers crossed that I still might make it.

We were asked to film a live slot for *Big Brother's Little Brother* and they quickly flashed up some sexy photographs of me. At this point I began to feel that they were using me, and warning bells began to ring inside my head. I stood at the back of the group and crouched on the floor, deciding that I did not want to play any part in this segment. Fortunately, it lasted just 15 minutes.

Now the countdown was under way.

The freak show had started, with drums rolling and lights flashing, and there was a ringmaster telling the members of the public who had poured in when to cheer and when to boo. And then Davina McCall appeared, looking like she wanted to be anywhere in the world but here.

Davina announced that *Big Brother* was about to start casting its vote. We were about to learn the identities of the housemates, and I knew, with absolute certainty, that I wasn't going to be one of them,

First in was a woman who ran a chicken farm, then a legless former soldier. And then a host of lookalikes – one after another. I was bored by now, and briefly considered showing my 'Spank Me' knickers to the cameras. I thought it might liven up proceedings.

It took an eternity for them to name everybody who was going in. And then, finally, for me and for the others who didn't get in, it was over. Around me, people were crying and stomping around in disgust and then the producers said they wanted to film us all – they begged me, but by then I'd had enough. I'd had more than enough, and I was out of there, just as fast as my little legs would carry me.

And do you know what? I am glad, really glad, that they didn't select me. In the aftermath of it all, somebody sold some ancient topless photos of me to the *Daily Star* – I wouldn't have minded so much, but if they had asked me, I would happily have let them take some new ones. Apart from anything else, I look better now.

CHAPTER 25
A Beastly Experience

I got a phone call asking if I was interested in appearing in a television series called *Beauty And The Beast* – the idea was that somebody like me, for whom appearance and beauty mean everything, would spend time sharing the life of an individual who, for whatever reason, looked ugly. It could have been that they were born with a facial disfigurement, or that they had suffered horrific injuries in a car crash or whatever.

I thought long and hard before saying yes, but the moment that the programme was announced, the media pounced on it, saying that it was exploiting people who had already suffered badly enough without being held up as freaks. What the media always tend to forget is that nobody ever forces anybody to appear in a TV series – they could always say no.

It wasn't long before I was left wishing that I had done precisely that.

Appropriately enough, *Beauty And The Beast* turned out to be what I can only describe as car crash TV.

For once, I should probably start at the end. After being away from my family for four days, I was on my way home to be reunited with Tony and Poppy. I should say that the make-up department had been to work on me beforehand, creating what appeared to be the most hideously ugly old woman. Even I had barely been able to look at myself in the mirror. God knows how my family were going to react.

My time away from Tony, Hannah and Poppy had brought it home to me just how obsessed we are with beauty – us as a society and, yes, me an individual. Vanity is a terrible thing, I now realise that.

As the car neared my home in Cambridgeshire, I struggled to fight back the tears that were welling up in my eyes. I was so looking forward to a cuddle and a kiss from the people who meant the world to me.

As I knocked on the front door, with the film crew in the background, Tony's face said it all. He was repulsed by the sight that greeted him. Yes, he tried to fight it, but he couldn't – and that, sadly, is the way that most of us react when greeted by ugliness. And yet we all want to take a sneaky look. It is hard not to stare when you see somebody in the street who is deformed.

I prayed that Poppy had gone to bed, that she would not be up to see what had become of me...

Beauty And The Beast was made by the Betty TV production company, it was screened in January 2011 and it probably provoked more of a reaction than anything else I have ever done – and that is saying something.

I 'starred', if that is the correct word, in an episode that was filmed at the end of August into the beginning of September 2010. The producers told me it would be a life-changing event, and they weren't wrong.

They had explained that I would be immersed in somebody else's life, somebody who would be as different from me as it was possible to be. Even I realised straight away that it had to be something to do with my looks – and if they were going to be asking me to share somebody else's life then it must surely mean that I would be meeting somebody who had suffered some sort of horrific facial injury.

Betty had already been to my home and filmed what they regarded as my typical life, a life that revolved around me trying to look my best at all times. And why shouldn't I? My face is, after all, my fortune.

The producers christened me 'Lady Burge', and it was obvious that they believed I lived a pampered lifestyle which, in many respects, is true. Of course they went out of their way to make me look like a spoilt little madam, too, filming me swinging around on my dancing pole and making sure that Tony was filmed while cooking dinner. I tried to make it clear that Tony enjoyed cooking the dinner, but it is not the conventional family scene, is it? Ah well, I figured that was why they had approached me in the first place. If I was just a normal woman, living a normal life, I wouldn't make good TV now, would I? Of course not.

They also made sure that they got Poppy to say that she preferred me without any make-up. Why? Because it meant that it got her out the door quicker in the morning when I took her to school.

Tony was encouraged to have his say, too, making it clear that he felt he lived with a mad woman, and that I was addicted to cosmetic surgery. It was all just for the cameras, of course, but it was exactly what they wanted to hear.

And they finished off the scene in my home by filming me applying a bit of filler to my face. They had captured it perfectly – 'Real Life Barbie', at home with her husband and young daughter, being waited on hand and foot. It was all bollocks, of course, but what harm could it do?

Day One:

I was taken to 35 Belgrave Square, London, not far from where Lady Thatcher lives. What a house it was, like something out of *Upstairs, Downstairs*. Or at least that was how it appeared at first. In fact, it was a pretty rundown affair, and I wasn't happy about sleeping in it.

But I didn't have time to think about that because they wanted me to get down to work straight away, and work involved walking into a room full of mirrors. I was told to stop at each one and preen and poke myself. It felt a bit like *Alice Through The Looking Glass*. There were mirrors of all shapes and sizes – high ones, small ones, tall ones, wide ones, narrow ones, cancave mirrors, convex mirrors. Every shape you could possibly imagine, and I was told to go completely over the top as I came to each one. I was happy to oblige.

The director told me to blow kisses at myself – God, how awful did that look? And then I had to stand in front of the final mirror and admire my backside.

On the count of five, they told me to turn round and wait. I was about to be confronted by my match for the week. The woman who confronted me took my breath away. I don't really know what I had expected – maybe I thought they would pair me up with a woman who had piled on the weight and let herself go?

No. The woman I found myself face to face with suffered the most grotesque facial disfigurement I had ever seen and I could feel my bottom lip quiver as I looked at her. I didn't want to look at her. I didn't want to stare. I wanted to look away, as quickly as possible.

She looked like she belonged in some circus freak show, and it brought back to me memories of the time when I had worked in Harley Street, helping women to cover scars and various forms of disfigurement. But nothing, and I do mean nothing, that I saw in Harley Street had prepared me for this. I admit it – I felt uncomfortable, and didn't know what to so, what to do or where to look.

I was told that her name was Susan, and I greeted her with a hug. At that moment, the programme's shrink walked in. Her name was Lachme, but I ended up calling her Lucky because I couldn't pronounce it.

Lucky welcomed us both to the 'beauty asylum' and informed us that we were going to dissect what beauty was, and what it meant to each one of us.

I admitted how important my looks were to me, and to everything that I did. Then I spoke about my lust for life and about how much I enjoyed sex and passion, and how they helped me to function as the person that I am. And being me, I tried to inject some humour into the situation.

Lucky asked why I'd had so much cosmetic surgery and I told her about being beaten up by a man who supposedly loved me, leaving me desolate and disfigured and struggling to cope with life. I was then told that I would be given a task to perform and that I was expected to do it properly, and with passion.

They did not allow Susan and I to connect or to get to know one another on our own terms – that would not have been good TV, would it?

Finally, they put us together again at dinner and told us to discuss society's preoccupation with celebrity and beauty. I admit that I spoke candidly about beauty, saying that we all wanted to look our best, and that nobody would consciously want to look awful. I stressed that I had experience of both sides of the coin, but the programme-makers clearly did not want me to dwell on my disfigurement. Oh no, the emphasis was to be on Susan and the way that the public perceived the way that she looked.

Susan told me her story, and it was awful. At the age of four months, doctors discovered that she had cancer and concluded that extensive radiation treatment was the only way to save her life. It killed the cancer, but it also took away half of her face and stunted this poor woman's growth. The press had said that this was going to be a freak show, and I now realised that they were absolutely right.

I tried to explain that Susan's story and mine were not dissimilar, but nobody was listening to me. Yes, I had been put together again, but I had also suffered years of mental and physical anguish – and even after all the surgery, I was still being branded as a freak.

When I said that more could be done to help Susan's appearance, and that there had been huge advances in plastic surgery in recent years, nobody was listening. They didn't want to hear it. I wondered what the following day would bring, and before we went to our bedrooms I gave Susan a little gift and a card – nothing special, just something to mark our meeting and the adventure we were about to embark upon.

Before I could go to sleep, I needed a glass of wine to settle my nerves, and the crew were happy enough to open a bottle of white for me. I then returned to my room, which contained a horrible single bed and all those bloody mirrors. Poppy had given me a toy bunny and I cuddled up to it, hoping to get a good night's sleep. In the end, I tossed and turned all night long and was still wide awake when they got me out of bed at 6am and then made sure I was fully made-up before the day unfolded.

Day Two:

The idea was to get Susan to embrace a day in the life of Sarah Burge, but it was so far removed from reality as to be absolutely absurd. All that they wanted to do was to portray me a vain air-head who was obsessed with beauty and celebrity.

We were taken to a London beauty salon, where I explained to Susan the various treatments I performed on myself on a regular basis. Nobody could argue with the benefits – yes, I might be a little bit vain, but the reality is that my skin is in pretty good nick for a woman of 50, and I am proud of that. Why wouldn't I be?

I took comfort from the fact that the programme would demonstrate that I had been doing something right for all these years.

They stripped my face of make-up in order to carry out a skin peel – I was happy to go along with all of this just as long as I could explain the benefits to Susan. They wanted to give her a skin peel too, but I made it clear that as far as I was concerned what she would really benefit from was plastic surgery. A skin peel would not address her problems in any way.

In the end, she had a micro-dermabrasion procedure which did actually make her skin look better and left her feeling better too. Perhaps my beauty treatments were not so bad after all?

Then the crew announced that they were going to put me through a photo shoot. I explained that, in my everyday life, I would never have a photo shoot done just for the sake of it. If I was having my photo taken, it might be for my autobiography, or it might be to accompany a newspaper or magazine article, or it might be to go along with the raunchy videos we make.

The producers didn't want to know.

"We just want a fashion shoot Sarah, with you looking glamorous."

"Bit I have never done a fashion shoot in my life, so it wouldn't be realistic. You would not be showing the real Sarah Burge; you would be showing the image you want to portray.

By now, Susan was saying that I was no longer the person she had met the day before, that I had turned into somebody else. What she was seeing was a woman who was prepared to stand up for herself. Why should I go along with this when it is not what I do and it is not who I am? In the end, I grew so frustrated that I ended up bursting into tears. I knew how this was panning out, and it did not take a genius to figure that it wasn't working out well for me.

I felt that I had been stripped of both my dignity and my profession-alism, and when those have gone, what else is left?

To make matters worse, Susan decided that she wanted to join in the fashion shoot and ended up trying on all the designer clothes that had been brought in for me to wear. She complained that none of them looked right on her, which was hardly surprising – and finally decided to pop on a little black number of her own.

The photographer then instructed her to pose this way and that, and my feelings of unease only grew as it began to look like I was trying to make a fool of her in my environment. Strangely, as the day wore on it was Susan who changed.

She began to boss me about – there is no other way to put it.

Susan then announced that she knew all about photo shoots, and that this was by no means the first she had ever done. I was staggered when she began to direct the crew and give them instructions, insisting that they show her all the photographs so that she could choose the ones to be displayed on the big screen. I found all of this very odd, especially as this was meant to be looking at a typical day in my life, but I had become the forgotten person, and it began to occur to me that maybe Susan had a huge chip on her shoulder because of the way she looked.

She had told me earlier that the crew were encouraging her to be nasty to me, and said that she was having none of it, but as time wore on, the temper and tantrums began.

The day wore on, and I hated it. But we still had an eventful evening in front of us. I had been told not to drink, but that was like a red rag to a bull, and I ended up grabbing a wine bottle far earlier than I would ever do under normal circumstances. In my defence, I felt that everything was out of control, and I could already imagine how the media would have a field day with it when it was broadcast.

So yes, I had a drink. It seemed obvious to me, even at this point, that they were looking to set me up as some kind of scapegoat, that they were looking to hang me and my reputation out to dry. I was Sarah Burge, the woman who'd had all the plastic surgery, the woman who ran celebrity parties and had a sexy alter ego called Madame Pink. I was Sarah Burge, the woman who attracted bad press for giving her teenage daughter botox and for teaching her youngest daughter how to pole dance – never mind the fact that I didn't actually teach her how to pole dance at all, and that is was all just a little bit of fun that once again got way out of hand and was blown up out of all proportion by the tabloids.

We had been told that we were going out on the town and that I had to wear something that was typical of my wardrobe, so ended up wearing a silver metallic dress that barely covered my backside, together with a flashing head-piece that looked like it belonged in Star Trek or Dr Who.

Susan was staring at me in disbelief as I slapped on more make-up and announced that the dress I was wearing represented everything I stood for in the beauty stakes – as far as I was concerned, I was just ahead of my time. And sometimes, you just have to give them what you think they want to hear. Through gritted teeth, she said: "I love your dress." Her eyes were saying: "I hate your dress – it makes you look like a slut."

And so we were put in a taxi and headed off to a bar in Piccadilly. As we got out of the taxi, passers-by stopped and stared – the two of us looked like the stars of a freak show. How appropriate. Some people wanted to take photos of us with their camera phones, but I was once again feeling very uncomfortable about the whole thing. Before I knew what was going on, we were surrounded by a group of drunken, jeering yobs who were poking fun at Susan's appearance. I wanted to punch them in the face. Instead, I grabbed her arm and we went into the bar.

As I ordered champagne, I told Susan that this was the type of place I would come to in order to relax after a busy day of meetings in London. She didn't seem interested, and after the way the yobs had treated her outside, I wasn't surprised.

The crew had told us just to sit and talk, and I did my best, in between glasses of champagne. Susan didn't drink, so I ended up throwing hers down my neck too.

During our conversation, I discovered that Susan had a sense of humour not unlike my own, so perhaps we were connecting after all? I told her that I knew many of the country's leading plastic surgeons and I said that I would happily take her to see them so that she could an expert opinion on what could be done to help her. She didn't seem to be too interested, and I began to get a horrible sinking feeling.

Yes, I felt desperately sorry for Susan. The way she looked, through no fault of her own, was awful, and I cannot imagine what it must have been like for her, but I was trying to offer help and encouragement, and all that I was getting back in return was a negative response. It made me feel thoroughly depressed.

The night ended with Susan singing the praises of all the high-end beauty products she was using. I couldn't believe what I was hearing – she didn't need beauty products or skin creams, she needed a new face!

I went to bed wearing a pair of "Spank Me" knickers, and that just about summed up how I felt.

Day Three:

This was the day when I had to step into Susan's shoes and find out what it was like to be her. I wasn't certain that I wanted to find out, but I had come this far, so there was no going back.

Not only hadn't I slept again, but I had also managed to pick up an eye infection so had to pile on the eye make-up to try and hide it. Susan told me that I wore too much make-up. Surprise! Surprise!

But before we could go any further, each of us had to sit on the couch for a touch of psycho-analysis. I went first. There was a screen in front of me, with members of my family being asked to give their views about what they thought of me and my beauty regime. First of all, pictures of me were flashed on the screen – schoolgirl Sarah, bunny girl Sarah, pole dancer Sarah. It was all so predictable.

And then, there was Tony on the screen announcing that I was "totally mad", and that I was addicted to plastic surgery. Poppy appeared to say that she preferred me without make-up, but it is amazing what you can do with a bit of clever editing.

Then it was Susan's turn, and there were only good things said about her. "Fabulous." "Amazing." "Fantastic." What a brain this woman had, but let's get something straight here and now – life had been incredibly cruel to Susan, and she had no choice but to channel all her efforts and energy into pursuing an academic career, because anything that involved her looks was never going to be a realistic option.

I was open-mouthed as she then accused me of calling her an "ugly minger" and stormed off the set. If they were trying to make me look like a monster, they were succeeding. What I had actually said was nobody in their mind would choose to be "ugly and minging", and I also added that of course I couldn't know what it must feel like to have the sort of disfigurement Susan had. That is very different from describing her as an "ugly minger". Why did nobody want to listen when I tried to explain how I had felt when I was beaten up? Why did nobody care about the pain and suffering and feelings of repulsion I felt when I had looked in a mirror? And why would nobody listen when I tried to explain to them that during my time working in Harley Street, I had gone out of my way to try and help people with facial disfigurements?

Susan told me that I couldn't possibly know what it was like to be her. In the end, I'd had enough and ended up in a heap, crying like a baby.

This, I am sure, is what they had wanted from the start. Well, now they had it.

The crew called a break, but not to see whether I was all right. No, they wanted to make sure that Susan had not been traumatised. By now, I was beginning to feel that I really would need to see a shrink when this was all over.

We were soon back in front of the cameras, being asked to summarise the day's events. I grabbed the bunny rabbit Poppy had given me and rocked backwards and forwards in floods of tears.

But still my misery wasn't over.

I was told to dress casually for Susan's night out. That wasn't difficult because the way I felt and looked I wasn't in the least bit interested in making any effort to get dressed up. My eyes and face were puffy from all the crying, and last thing I wanted to do was to go out, but I had to go along with it.

Our car pulled up outside a pub, and I had to wait for my cue to walk in. All sorts of things were going through my mind as I waited outside, but my biggest dread was that I walk into the pub and find it full of people with disfigured faces.

It was almost as bad. This was a spit-and-sawdust pub, with an old man in the corner playing the piano. Somebody gave me a glass of wine and then Susan stood up and started singing. Not only that, but she started singing really, really well. Remember the way that the nation reacted to Susan Boyle's first TV appearance? This affected me in much the same way. And before long, everybody in the pub was joining in.

And then came the dreaded words. "You are up next Sarah," said Susan. Me? You have got to be joking. Ah well, in for a penny, in for a pound. Thank God for my theatre training, because I had learnt a few music hall numbers in my time and I was soon belting them out for all I was worth – and the more I had to drink, the more I enjoyed it.

When the singing was over, I was "interviewed" on the street outside, and asked how amazing I thought Susan's voice was. Surely I must have been impressed with all the talents that she possessed? Well I was hardly going to say no, was I?

On the way back to the house we decided to stop for a kebab, which I ordered in Arabic. Amazingly, nobody asked me how I knew the language. I quietly reassured myself with the knowledge that there was only one day to go.

I had thought that this was going to be a journey of exploration for two people, but that was never going to be the case – this was always just a trip for one person.

Day Four:

On the final day, all that I was interested in doing was counting down the hours until I got home, but they weren't finished with me yet.

Because Susan had stormed off the day before, we still had to complete her day, so were taken to Oxford Street so that people could stop and stare at her and she could talk about she was discriminated against when it came to finding a job.

Perhaps she was applying for the wrong sort of job? I pointed out that it was against the law to discriminate against people on the grounds of a disability, but Susan wasn't having any of that.

The whole Oxford Street experience was very uncomfortable. The point of it was to get people to stare, and to record their reactions, but it seemed pretty obvious to me that if you turned up in any busy street with a film crew then people would stop and stare. I felt like a freak – again.

Then we had to go into Harvey Nicholls, where Susan started pulling clothes from the rails, telling me this dress would suit me, and I should buy that top. I don't know why, but she seemed to have got it into her head that I liked shopping, but it is actually one of my least favourite things to do. So I sat down on a chair and fell asleep.

We were interviewed again, and I made it perfectly clear that I hadn't enjoyed the experience, that I had found Susan to be quite a domineering woman at times, and that was something that I couldn't quite get my head around.

But still it wasn't over. During my final debrief from the programme's shrink, she announced that I needed to face up to my greatest fears, and to do that they were going to age me by at least 20 years, using make-up and prosthetics. "Great," I though. "This will be a perfect reminder of how I am never going to allow myself to look."

I had to stand in front of the camera and remove my eyelashes and all my make-up, while Susan declared that I looked much prettier and kinder without it. Naturally, I wasn't allowed anywhere near a mirror while they set about the ageing process. Eventually, when they were finished, I was allowed to look. I let out a moan, but I don't know whether it was because of what I was looking at or because I was simply so exhausted.

They told me that I was going to have to face the world as a 70-year-old, so they took me to Victoria station to record the public's reaction. There was no reaction. I was invisible. I felt old and depressed – even my personality seemed to drain away.

The producers told me that they wanted me to leave the show and return home as this anonymous old woman, but first they wanted me to sum up what impact the programme had had on me. I told them that, for the first time in four days, Susan and I had connected – I now looked old, tired and ugly, and her attitude towards me had changed. I hated to be cruel but, as far as I was concerned, this said far more about her than it did about me. She was the one who was narrow minded and suffered from prejudices, not me.

And then it was home, praying Poppy was in bed. I hadn't been allowed to forewarn Tony that I was returning as a 70-year-old woman. They wanted to record the shock on his face. I knocked on the door and he answered – it took him a few seconds, but then it registered that it was me who was standing in front of him and he looked stunned. The crew tried to persuade him that looks are in the eye of the beholder and that he should love me for who I am – but he does love me for who I am. And in any event, I would seriously worry about him if he had found me more attractive as a 70-year-old woman than he does when all that crap was stripped off.

It was a beastly experience, but it left me feeling at the end of it all that I am happy in my own skin, and that I just want to be me. Whoever that may be.

I met up with Susan for some catch-up interviews and after spending some quality time in her company I realised that I could actually have some fun with her. The two of us formed a bond, exchanged telephone numbers and we now talk on the phone from time to time.

I am not going to tell you that we will ever be best friends, but we do respect one another and recognise our differences. In truth, I am glad that I met Susan.

CHAPTER 26
Into The Bear Pit

I have always refused to appear on the *Jeremy Kyle Show*. There have been several opportunities for me to do so, but as much as I enjoy being in the limelight, I draw the line at Kyle.

I just don't like the way that he treats people. He talks to many of his guests as if they were something he had just stepped in – yes, it's true that some pretty unsavoury characters appear on the show, and it could be argued that they get nothing more or less than they deserve.

My feeling was always that if I agreed to do one of his shows, he would do everything within his power to make me look like a freak, so why would I want to put myself in that position?

During the late summer of 2010 I was asked if I would like to appear on a programme looking at the whole question of cosmetic surgery, and I readily agreed to do so. The idea was that there was going to be a panel of experts and the whole issue would be debated. I knew that word 'debate' would mean that I would inevitably find myself in the firing line, but so what? We didn't know who was going to be hosting it, but I had been given the impression that it was going to be fronted by Peaches Geldof.

A researcher phoned me several times, and it became increasingly obvious to me that they were desperate to get me on the show. It eventually emerged that Peaches was not going to be presenting it, and I kept asking who was going to replace her. Eventually the researcher told me that it was going to be Jeremy Kyle because they had been unable to find anybody else.

As soon as I heard that, I told her that I wouldn't do the programme, but she was very persuasive, telling me that I would just be one person on a panel of professionals who would be debating the benefits of plastic surgery. She assured me that it wasn't the Jeremy Kyle Show – it was a medical show, looking at serious issues, with Kyle acting as the host. Even then, I still had serious reservations about agreeing to appear but she eventually persuaded me, assuring me that everything was going to be just fine.

Agreeing to do it turned out to be one of the biggest mistakes of my life.

Right from the start, Kyle attacked me. Within the first 60 seconds I was asked if I was prostitute and whether I had sex with men for money. He basically accused me of being a freak and saying that I was a shallow person. What the hell any of that had to do with plastic surgery is anybody's guess.

Kyle and his producer knew that I had been a victim of domestic abuse and were fully aware that this was why I'd had plastic surgery in the first place, but no mention was made of that.

The worst thing about it was that he would make a point or ask a question and then not give me the opportunity to answer. It was awful.

I was verbally abused and bullied by this man. I find it ironic when I watch his shows and sometimes hear him suggesting to guests that they need to attend anger management courses – my perception is that it is Mr Kyle who would benefit from such a course.

I worry that somebody will end up committing suicide after appearing on one of his shows. Personally, I was so shocked by his verbal onslaught upon me that I could barely breathe. I didn't know what to say or do and couldn't think straight.

Worse than that, in the aftermath of appearing on the show, I began to suffer flashbacks and nightmares that brought my ordeal at Faisal's hands back to life once again. With every insult that he threw at me, the studio audience cheered louder and louder. These people knew nothing about me or my life. They hadn't the first idea what I had been through, and it was horrible to sit there knowing that every single one of them was against me.

Afterwards, I reported Kyle's verbal assault to the police. As far as I had been concerned, I was in a place of work, and nobody should have to endure this kind of thing while at work. Bullying in the workplace is not tolerated anywhere, but, much my disappointment, the police decided to take no further action.

I told the producers of the programme that I was considering taking out an injunction to prevent them from broadcasting the show and although I will never know whether or not this had any impact upon them, they did eventually tell me that they were not going to screen the programme.

It was another lesson learnt.

I have made many television appearances, especially since the tabloids christened me 'Real-Life Barbie'. Some of them have been fun, some of them have been excruciating and on some of them I have felt that I have been hauled in front of the cameras in order to be humiliated.

Let's start with *Richard And Judy*, the Channel 4 tea-time show. They were having a discussion on cosmetic surgery and I was asked to appear. They were responding to a piece that had appeared following a woman who was trying to have cosmetic surgery done abroad, but on a budget of only about £4,000.

She had a tummy tuck that was filmed, and they wanted me on the programme as an expert. Their chauffeur picked us up from the station and we duly arrived at the studio, where we were greeted by a runner who ushered me in to have my hair and make-up done.

I always get the impression with these programmes that they do everything within their power to make you look as awful as possible. The make-up girl swept my hair across one side of my face – it was hideous.

Also on with me was the journalist Amanda Platell, who quite clearly was never going to be on my side, and there was the woman who been on the plastic surgery quest.

It was a live show, and I liked that because it meant that they couldn't edit it. So the conversation began. The woman who had been operated on was asked to talk through the procedure while pictures of it were shown, and Richard and Judy made a big play of saying how horrible it all was, and how difficult it was to watch. Remember that this was going out while people were sitting down to eat their dinners.

Platell then had her say, but nobody was paying a blind bit of notice of me – it was as if I was there for decorative purposes, and that didn't suit me at all. I was ready to walk off the set, and finally Richard turned to me and said: "Sarah, don't you think that what you have done to yourself is self-mutilation?"

I wanted to tell him to stop being such an arse-hole. Instead, I looked him straight in the eye and replied: "I really wish that I could frown at what you have just said [I had just had some botox injections, so frowning was not a possibility]. You don't expect me to give that question a sensible answer, do you?"

Platell then wanted to know how old I was and why I'd had so much plastic surgery done. I told her that I had it done because I wanted to look good, and muttered under my breath that it was because I didn't to look like her. It was the truth. I didn't want to look like her and I didn't want to look like Judy. They had been horrible to me, and I gave them what I thought they deserved. If they had treated me properly, I would have answered their questions properly.

It was the last show of the series and afterwards there was a party. My first inclination was to storm off home, but I figured that Tony and I may as well see what we could get out of Channel 4. As I was standing there, Amanda Platell wandered over and asked me who had performed my surgery because she was thinking of having some done herself.

So she had sat in front of the cameras and announced that she would never have anything done, that anybody who did was insecure, but the moment the cameras stopped rolling, she was all over me for information on good plastic surgeons. I was stunned. And so was Tony.

Ricky Gervais had been on the show and he was also at the party. I have no feelings either way about his ability to make people laugh – I can take him or leave him. But I could not believe the way that everybody was fawning around him, telling him how wonderful he was, asking whether he wanted anything. It was sickening.

As for Richard and Judy, they snubbed us totally. It would have cost nothing for either of them to have a word with me, but no. Richard spoke to Amanda Platell, to Gervais and to the woman who'd had the surgery, but it was as if I didn't exist.

Afterwards I received hundreds of emails supporting the approach that I had taken.

On the other hand, I was treated with nothing but respect by Andrew Castle, Penny Smith and Ben Shepherd when I appeared on *GMTV* to discuss bum implants. Penny Smith had a bit of a reputation for being difficult to work with, but I found her to be a really genuine person who was interested in what I had to say, and who listened.

Then there was the *Maury Povich Show* in the United States – it is a similar format to *The Jeremy Kyle Show*, where they wheel out a host of low-lifes who want to know if they have really fathered the child that their wife has just given birth to. Maury shouts at them and then produces the DNA results, and shouts some more.

But I figured that I could hold my own against him in a plastic surgery special, especially as they were prepared to pay me plenty to appear. For one day's work, they paid me about £8,000, and they also paid to fly Tony and Poppy out with me, and then put us up in a fabulous hotel, and paid for all our meals.

The day before the programme, one of their runners came out to the hotel where they had put us up to make sure that everything was okay, and that we were happy with the accommodation and the food. He then explained exactly what would happen the following day.

We were taken for some filming before going to the studio. There were numerous other programmes being filmed, and I couldn't believe some of the stuff I heard – people who were appearing on the likes of *The Jerry Springer Show* were being coached in the art of crying and expressing shock. The whole bloody thing was stage managed. They had to cry on order, and had to throw their arms in the air at the right moment, to get the maximum possible impact.

"What have they got in store for me?" I wondered. I didn't have to wait long to find out. They sat me down and told me what they wanted me to say.

"So you don't want me just to answer the questions that Maury asks me?"

"No, no, no. That is not the way it works."

I wasn't desperately happy but I figured that as long as they were paying me, then I would go along with whatever they wanted. I was even told when to stop and pause, when to sigh, when to be dramatic. I was told that when I walked out on stage I had to wave both arms at the audience and wiggle my backside before sitting down beside Maury.

The show was filmed in front of a New York audience that had been worked up into a frenzy beforehand, but one of the things you have to understand is that many American women aspire to have plastic surgery as appearance is everything in the States.

I couldn't quite bring myself to wave the way they wanted, but I did my best, and took my seat as instructed. Why they gave me a script I had no idea, because Maury would not let anybody get a word in. It was his show. In fact, all around the building there had been cardboard cut-outs of him. I thought it was very funny.

To be fair to him, Maury was trying to have a serious debate about cosmetic surgery, which would have been absolutely fine had he given anybody who knew anything about the subject an opportunity to have their say, but as hard as I tried, he wouldn't let me speak and I couldn't take it seriously.

In the end, I tried to laugh and joke with him, and he said: "Well Sarah, you are obviously a very happy lady."

And do you know what? I rather think that I am.

After everything that I have been through in my life, I consider myself incredibly fortunate to have hooked up again with Tony, and to have a daughter with him was just amazing. Numerous people have approached me from America suggesting that my story would make an amazing movie – I am sure that it would, although I don't know if anybody would believe it.